Born in Glasgow, Ro̶ up with a passion fo̶ ̶e̶s̶. Choosing medicine a̶ ̶from Glasgow University in 1̶ ̶ne next three years as a psychiatris̶ ̶my. From 1953 to 1956 he worked at th̶ ̶Royal Mental Hospital and then at Glasgow U̶ ̶y̶. *Wisdom, Madness and Folly* (1985) gives a vivid pic̶ure of a stimulating, if emotionally ambivalent, upbringing and the early years of his professional life. It was during this time that he came to question the power relationship between mental patients and their doctors, and the received wisdom of locked wards and chemical or electroshock therapy. From 1957 to 1961 he worked at the Tavistock Clinic in London and went on to set out his radical ideas about the nature of mental disturbance in *The Divided Self* (1960), *Self and Others* (1961) and *Sanity, Madness and the Family* (1964). These works resisted definitions of 'mental illness' in favour of understanding schizophrenia as 'a special strategy that a person invents in order to live in an unlivable situation.' Laing's approach saw mental disturbance in relation to the sufferer's immediate family and the abnormal stresses of modern society, and he set both within the wider and more philosophical contexts of personal alienation and existential crisis.

He was director of the Langham Clinic in London (1962–5), a member of the Tavistock Institute for Human Relations, chairman of the Philadelphia Association (1964–82) and a fellow of the Foundations Fund for Research in Psychiatry. His ideas were put into practice in 1965 at Kingsley Hall in London, which he helped to found as a community where 'patients' and 'doctors' lived together as equals.

Laing's ideas were to become associated with hippy

excess in the 1970s, something that his later lifestyle and his interest in psychedelic experience did little to refute. But the truly humane force of his work derived from his philosophical and creative interests and what we would now call a poststructuralist sense of the human subject and the unstable condition of even the healthiest among us. His many writings include *The Politics of Experience and the Bird of Paradise* (1967), *The Politics of the Family* (1976), *The Voice of Experience* (1982), as well as the semantic entanglements of *Knots* (1970) and the poems of *Sonnets* (1980).

R. D. LAING
WISDOM, MADNESS AND FOLLY

The Making of a Psychiatrist
1927–57

Introduced by
CRAIG BEVERIDGE &
RONALD TURNBULL

CANONGATE
CLASSICS
89

First published in 1985 by MacMillan London Ltd. This edition first published as a Canongate Classic in 1998 by Canongate Books, 14 High Street, Edinburgh EH1 1TE. Copyright © R. D. Laing, 1985. Introduction copyright © Craig Beveridge and Ronald Turnbull 1998.

The publishers gratefully acknowledge general subsidy from the Scottish Arts Council towards the Canongate Classics series and a specific grant towards the publication of this volume.

Set in 10pt Plantin by Hewer Text Ltd, Leith. Printed and bound by Caledonian, Bishopbriggs, Scotland.

Canongate Classics
Series Editor: Roderick Watson
Editorial board: J. B. Pick, Cairns Craig,
Dorothy McMillan

British Library Cataloguing in Publication Data
A catalogue record for this book is available on request from the British Library.

ISBN 0 86241 831 3

Contents

Introduction

Ronald Laing's intellectual status and achievement defy straightforward classification. By training and profession a psychiatrist and psychoanalyst, he also experimented in alternative approaches to the treatment of mental suffering. He could, then, be placed alongside figures such as Suttie, Fairbairn and Sutherland, in that still-to-be-written work on the broader cultural significance of Scottish psychiatry and psychoanalysis.

But this would do justice neither to the range of Laing's major interests – which included philosophy and theology as well as psychology – nor to the impact of his ideas. He owed his fame to writing which challenged psychiatric doctrine and practice on broad theoretical and ethical grounds, a critique which placed him, in the public eye at least, among the revolutionary theorists (Marcuse, Fanon *et al.*) of '6os New Leftism; and his publications included an expository book on the philosophy of Sartre. We might call him a philosopher, though not in conventional academic terms; or a social and cultural critic; or, quite simply, a thinker. In any case, whatever label is attached, this 'manifestly remarkable' man – as he struck one acquaintance – is an outstanding figure in recent Scottish cultural history.

Commentary on Laing's ideas – like the Fontana *Modern Masters* volume devoted to him – has often disregarded the cultural background, as if his work had materialized out of nothing and nowhere; and such neglect is encouraged by prominent social history texts which depict the kind of milieu in which Laing grew up as a cultural void, a 'world of

deprivation', in the words of one famous historian. The pages
in *Wisdom, Madness and Folly* on Laing's Glasgow childhood
in the 1930s serve to reveal the inaccuracy of such representa-
tions. (This is not to overlook the obvious point that memoirs,
like other histories, cannot be judged in terms of a simple
binary logic of truth or falsehood; aspects may be forgotten,
downplayed or suppressed, or exaggerated – the case, it has
been suggested, of Laing's negative account of his mother's
behaviour in this autobiography.)

Laing's thought has to be traced – where else? – to its
roots in his social and cultural formation. Or in more
rigorous terms, which we borrow from the social theory
of Pierre Bourdieu, crucial explanatory weight is borne by
the 'habitus', the enduring set of codes and dispositions
and the 'system of generative schemes' acquired from the
socio-cultural environment. In early experience, Bourdieu
writes, 'the structures characterising a determinate class of
conditions of existence produce the structures of the habitus, which in their turn are the basis of the perception and
appreciation of all subsequent experiences . . .'. Thus the
habitus ensures 'the active presence of past experiences . . .
in the form of schemes of perception, thought and action . . .'. (Bourdieu, *The Logic of Practice*, 1990).

Laing's habitus, as *Wisdom, Madness and Folly* makes
clear, involved a strong religious moment. His childhood
and youth were an immersion in an evangelically-tinged
Presbyterianism: Sunday school from the age of four, the
catechism (quoted, significantly, at some length in the
text), memorisation of passages from the Bible, daily school
service, the Scripture Union and other Christian groups,
daily private prayer. Of course, you can leave the church.
Laing did. The church doesn't leave you.

In an essay published in *The Listener* in 1970, Laing
wrote:

> I grew up, theologically speaking, in the nineteenth
> century: lower-middle-class Lowland Presbyterianism,

corroded by nineteenth-century materialism, scientific
rationalism and humanism . . . I remember vividly
how startled I was to meet for the first time, when I
was eighteen, people of my age who had never
opened a Bible . . . For the first time in my life, I
could see myself being looked at rather as I imagine a
native may see himself looked at by an attentive,
respectful anthropologist. I could see myself regarded
with incredulity by an eighteen-year-old French girl, a
student from the Sorbonne, as some idealistic
barbarian still occupied by issues of religious belief,
disbelief or doubt, still living before the
Enlightenment, exhibiting in frayed but still
recognisable form the primitive thought forms of the
savage mind.

The importance in Laing's development of the tension
indicated here between 'Lowland Presbyterianism' and
secular rationalism, between theological culture and *Auf-
klärung*, surfaces almost immediately in this memoir. At-
tempting to explain how he came to be at odds with
mainstream psychiatry, Laing recounts, discussing his early
career, his puzzlement that some psychiatrists regarded
Kierkegaard as mad. This was hardly a view Laing could
share; after all, his own roots were in a culture which would
pronounce mad, not Kierkegaard, but these psychiatrists.

Laing's first, and most influential book, *The Divided Self*,
was completed in 1957 and published in 1959, thus pre-
dating, incidentally, Michel Foucault's *Folie et déraison*, the
other text – later reviewed by Laing in enthusiastic terms –
which helped set in motion an important public debate
about psychiatric discourse and practice. Largely due to his
experience as a psychiatrist in the British army, recounted
in this book, Laing had already come to a Foucauldian-type
view that judgements about madness reflected as much the
operations of social and political power as a disinterested
search for medical and scientific truth.

The Divided Self is a remarkable achievement, not least
because it draws on philosophy and theology as well as
work in psychology, and because it is based on European
thinkers and traditions of thought – existentialism and
phenomenology; Kierkegaard, Heidegger, Husserl, Sartre.
This 'generalist' approach and the Continental-philosophi-
cal terms of reference, which reflect Laing's contacts with
Glasgow philosophical circles (as we sketch in more detail
below), were completely alien to the arid, insular Anglo-
British intellectual culture of the time. (One colleague at
the London Tavistock Clinic – John Bowlby – urged Laing
to excise from the text such terms as existential, phenom-
enological and ontological.)

Laing's critique of conventional psychiatry centred, as
Wisdom, Madness and Folly underlines, on the failure to
approach the patient as a locus of subjectivity, intentionality and agency, or, in other words, a *person* ('The "com-
mitteed" person,' Laing says in *The Politics of Experience* 'is
degraded from full existential and legal status as human
agent and responsible person . . . he is invalidated as a
human being . . .'). This is not only an ethical but an
epistemological failure. 'We shall be concerned,' Laing
writes, 'with people who experience themselves as automata, as robots, as bits of machinery, or even as animals.
Such persons are rightly regarded as crazy. Yet why do we
not regard a theory which seeks to transmute persons into
automata or animals as equally crazy?' Behind attempts to
account for human behaviour in chemical, mechanical and
purely biological terms lies the belief that only thus can
scientificity be attained. 'There is a common illusion that
one can somehow increase one's understanding of a person
if one can translate a personal understanding of him into
the impersonal terms of a sequence of it-processes.' But the
'objectivity' thus achieved is pseudo-scientific. Laing's
approach is to attend to the patient's intentionality, his/
her own conception of their being, and to his/her relations
with others. (One of the key ideas developed by Laing was

that mental 'illness' is the outcome of oppressive social relations, and especially of struggles for power within the family.)

More than anything else, Laing here insists, patients are simply human, like anyone else. The relationship between psychiatrist and patient must therefore be a personal one, centred on 'the original bond of I and You': the model of detached observation imported from natural science is misplaced. The aim is understanding rather than explanation – and 'for understanding one might say love'. *Wisdom, Madness and Folly* contains a moving account of how what he calls the 'spirit of fellowship' engendered by Hogmanay could transform even the most withdrawn of Laing's patients at Gartnavel.

If in his first book, then, Laing was opposing the illegitimate extension of natural scientific paradigms to the study of persons and interpersonal relationships, in a late and astonishing essay entitled 'What is the matter with mind?' (1980) he attacked the victory of a generalised positivist or scientistic ethos in much fiercer terms. Science, he says, ignores 'love and hate, joy and sorrow, misery and happiness, pleasure and pain, right and wrong, purpose, meaning, hope, courage, despair, God, heaven and hell, grace, sin, salvation, damnation . . .' (This is the return of Kierkegaard, with a vengeance!) Because of the successes and prestige of natural science, Laing wants to say, whole areas of human experience are devalorised: reality and objectivity are denied to all those phenomena present to consciousness which are not amenable to quantification and experimental control. 'All sensibility, all values, all quality, all feelings, all motives, all intentions, spirit, soul, consciousness, subjectivity: almost everything, in fact, which we ordinarily take to be real is de-realized, is stripped of its pretensions to reality', and the conviction spreads that 'all our subjective values are objectively valueless'.

Understanding, Gadamer writes in *Wahrheit und Methode* (1960), is 'less to be thought of as a subjective act'

than 'as conscription into an event of tradition'. Laing is
not, as has often been assumed, an isolated figure in recent
Scottish intellectual history. An inclination to question the
claims of science (without, however, lapsing into any kind
of irrationalism); the concern with the threat posed to
ethics by the spread of positivist modes of thought; the
refusal to ignore or disesteem the dimensions of experience, reasoning and reality which are beyond the scope of
natural scientific knowledge; an insistence on the phenomenon of *personhood*, and concern about its fate in modern
cultural conditions – these attitudes and interests, as we
have argued elsewhere, link Laing to a number of other
recent Scottish thinkers, such as the theologians John
Baillie, Ronald Gregor Smith and John Macquarrie, and
the philosophers John Macmurray (an acknowledged influence) and C. A. Campbell (whose classes at Glasgow
Laing attended). This 'personalist' movement in Scotland
reflected a strong interest in the work of German and
Jewish thinkers, especially Martin Buber, whose importance to Laing can be seen in *Wisdom, Madness and Folly*.

It is worth noting, in this connection, that before moving
to London Laing was a member of a discussion group
which had a marked existentialist and personalist orientation. This was sometimes called the Abenheimer group or
Schorstein group, after its two Jewish members who had
settled in Glasgow. Gregor Smith (a Buber expert) and
Macquarrie were also members. Continental philosophy
and theology dominated the group's discussions, which
concerned, among others, Kierkegaard, Heidegger, Jaspers, Buber, Bultmann, Tillich, Sartre and Unamuno.
Laing read to the group drafts of parts of *The Divided Self*.
Joe Schorstein, who worked in Glasgow as a neuro-sur-
geon, was the only person Laing ever referred to as 'my
spiritual father'. Not only did they share the same interests
– music as well as European philosophy and theology:
Schorstein, the son of a Hasidic rabbi, had experienced
a spiritual trajectory similar to Laing's, and, like Laing, was

torn – as the opposition is stated in these pages – between 'the twin figures, for me, of Kierkegaard and Nietzsche, Christ and Anti-Christ, the knight of faith, the destiny of nihilism . . .'.

Laing was a major figure, whose place in the history of ideas is secure; at the same time, his work is a notable recent moment in a Scottish intellectual tradition, in its dialogue with European thought, in its refusal of limitation to specialist detail, in its theoretical grappling with fundamental human issues, and, not least, in the qualities of passion and humanity which so imbue this autobiography.

Craig Beveridge
Ronald Turnbull

None the less, he knew that the tale he had to tell could not be one of a final victory. It could only be the record of what had had to be done, and what assuredly would have to be done again in the never-ending fight against terror, and its relentless onslaughts, despite their personal afflictions, by all who, while unable to be saints, but refusing to bow down to pestilences, strive their utmost to be healers.

Albert Camus
La Peste

Author Introduction

In the last ten years or so, my destiny has taken me to many parts of the world where I have met old friends whom I have never met before. These are people who knew me from my books, and from reports of an experiment begun in 1964 in Kingsley Hall, a community centre in London, where several of us lived with a number of very disturbed 'psychotic' people who would otherwise have been in mental hospitals or psychiatric units and treated accordingly. Among us there were no staff, no patients, no locked doors, no psychiatric treatment to stop or change states of mind.

We declared a free-for-all: freedom to think, see, feel in any way whatever; freedom of biorhythm (autorhythm) for all of us. On the other hand, transgressive conduct for whatever reason, of whatever kind is objectionable. On this or any other issue we took our chances together.

Since this is in many respects the exact opposite of the usual psychiatric approach, it has come in for a lot of criticism, controversy, and misunderstanding.* I am often asked how I, as a psychiatrist, came to a point of view, right or wrong, about psychiatry that is so different from, and sometimes so at odds with, a great deal of the psychiatry in which I was trained.

This memoir is a response to such questions. It covers the first thirty years of my life, from 1927 to 1957. I am not trying to justify myself, or prove that I am right. I have tried

* There are, however, a number of places in Europe and America which now put this approach into play.

to depict aspects of my world, and of my reactions to it. There is nothing here about my sex or family life, little about friends and social life, almost nothing about theory, books, articles, scientific details. What is here are the sorts of things that 'struck' me on the road to seeing and responding to the suffering with which psychiatry is involved in a different way from the usual. This difference is not about scientific facts. As far as I am aware, I have never said that a scientific, clinical, medical fact is not exactly what it is: a scientific, clinical, medical fact. But one can see the same facts differently. One can construe them differently. So, here, I am trying to describe different points of view, and to show how I came to mine. No facts are in dispute. I believe that to give serious consideration to the issues that arise from seeing the same differently itself contributes to lessening some of the fear, pain, madness and folly in the world.

As a young psychiatrist in general hospitals and psychiatric hospitals, I administered locked wards and ordered drugs, injections, padded cells and straitjackets, electric shocks, deep insulin comas and the rest. I was uneasy about lobotomies but not sure why. Usually all this treatment was against the will of its recipients. I went around in a white coat, with stethoscope, tendon hammer and ophthalmoscope sticking out of my pockets, like any other doctor. Like them, I examined patients clinically. I had samples of blood, urine, spinal fluid sent for laboratory analysis, ordered electroencephalograms and so on.

It looked the same as the rest of medicine, but it was different. I was puzzled, and uneasy. Hardly any of my psychiatric colleagues seemed puzzled or uneasy. This made me even more puzzled and uneasy.

ONE

Psychiatry Today

PSYCHIATRY TODAY is a set of institutions within the network of medical institutions that extends over much of the world – Europe, the USA, the USSR, China, Australia, New Zealand, parts of South America, Africa, India, etc. In its theory, practice, functions, position and power, it is an integral part of these larger institutions. As medical students and young doctors, all prospective psychiatrists have to be steeped in medicine-as-a-whole before they can become psychiatrists. This medical training distinguishes psychiatrists from non-medical mental-health professionals. Many doctors are not psychiatrists, but there are no psychiatrists who are not doctors. One may cease to be a psychiatrist without ceasing to be a doctor. If one ceases to be a doctor, one ceases to be a psychiatrist.

The word 'psychiatry' was coined to refer to the institution of a discipline within medicine. Etymologically, the word means psychological healing in the sense of the science and art of healing the psyche, mind, soul, person. But psychiatry is in fact a branch of medicine. Medical psychiatry is one approach to the art of psychological healing. A mental healer may be a psychiatrist. A psychiatrist may or may not be a mental healer. A mental healer may be a priest, or a shaman. In cultures which are still not technologically developed, or destroyed, I have met several 'primitive' priests, shamans, medicine men who have medical qualifications. But this is very rare.

The art of non-medical psychiatric mental healing has

nothing to do with psychiatry, at present, though in future there may be more cross-fertilization.*

As a medical student (1945–51) I encountered no such rift within medical psychiatry itself. I was aware of psychiatry as a division of medicine, with several subdivisions itself: there were, as there are, different 'schools' or orientations within psychiatry. It took me some time to figure out the medical politics of these orientations – the biologic-organic, the dynamic, the social, the existential and so forth – and it took me several years to realize the extent to which 'psychiatry' as a whole is different from the rest of medicine. In some medical schools 'psychiatry' is taught to medical students virtually as neurology. Psychiatry is really neuropsychiatry, neuropsychiatry is really neuroscience. Psychiatry, neuropsychiatry and neurology are branches, basically, of biology (including genetics, biophysics and biochemistry) applied to medicine.

The term 'medicine' itself is tricky. It is sometimes used for the whole medical profession, for medicine-in-general, along with general surgery, obstetrics and gynaecology, public health, paediatrics, geriatrics, psycho-social medicine, neurology, dermatology, and specialties within specialties – neurosurgery, cardiac surgery, thanatology. As a branch of modern Western medicine, within the international medical community, psychiatry is often ranked alongside surgery, medicine, obstetrics and gynaecology as a major division of medicine-in-general, although in some places it is considered a division of a division, a branch of a branch (general medicine) of medicine in the overall sense. Psychiatry itself has subdivisions, from child psychiatry to psychogeriatrics,

---

* The term 'anti-psychiatry' was coined by the psychiatrist David Cooper because he felt that psychiatry as the theory and practice of medical psychiatry was and is predominantly repressive, anti-psychiatric in the sense of the science and art of mental healing. Quite a few medical psychiatrists agree with him.

and addresses itself in different ways to different domains – biologic, social, for example.

Psychiatry has many functions. Some of these are the same as those of other fields of Western medicine, but psychiatry is unique in several respects. It is the only branch of medicine that treats people physically in the absence of any known physical pathology. It is the only branch of medicine that 'treats' conduct, alone, in the absence of symptoms and signs of illness of the usual kind. It is the only branch of medicine that treats people against their will, in any way it likes, if it deems it necessary. It is the only branch of medicine that imprisons patients, if judged necessary.

What I seemed to be engaged in was a concerted effort to stop undesired states of mind and conduct, and to keep undesired people in such undesired states of mind and conduct away from people outside, who did not want them around. Italian psychiatrists have recently almost entirely given up offering this service. Can our society, as it exists, do without it? What alternative will emerge? Crisis intervention? But supposing an intolerable impasse remains? If a violinist in an orchestra is out of tune and does not hear it, and does not believe it, and will not retire, and insists on taking his seat and playing at all rehearsals and concerts and ruining the music, what can be done? If all persuasion fails, is there anything else to do than to have him or her removed, by physical force, against his or her will, and *kept away* for as long as he or she persists in spoiling the fun for everyone else, call him or her ill or not?

It is not easy. What do we do when we don't know what to do? I want that guy out of sight, out of sound, out of mind. I want to get on with the music. Fair enough? But how? What would we do without psychiatrists? If not psychiatrists, the police? The police are not rushing to volunteer to 'fill the gap'.

The situation keeps cropping up in our society, when, no matter how liked, esteemed or loved, some people become insufferable to others. No one they know wants to live with them. They are not breaking the law, but they arouse in those around them such urgent feelings of pity, worry, fear, disgust, anger, exasperation, concern, that something has to be done. A social worker or psychiatrist is 'brought in'. He or she is there to exercise discretion and responsibility in deciding what is to happen. The first, decisive, crunch decision is: should *this* person, or *that* person, be taken away, locked up, and observed for a while? Then comes the second decision: should this person be kept in for a further period of observation, maybe 'treated'? In Italy, where psychiatrists refuse to make these decisions, they are trying to develop the art of helping 'the group' to resolve the 'crisis' within itself. What are the ordinary limits of ordinary people? The 'need' for this removal, seclusion and treatment service is not manufactured by psychiatrists. There is a consumer demand. As long as there is, some group will be appointed to meet it. Such intervention may not always be controlled by doctors. It is difficult to imagine our society without such a service, run under the control of the medical profession or not.

There he sits. In a deserted office in inner London at ten o'clock on a Friday night. He does not move. He does not speak. He has been sitting like that for twelve hours. No one knows why. No one knows who he is. Hospital or prison? The police don't want him. Hospital it has to be. Hospital it is.

The offender or intruder is taken away to a locked ward. He is observed. He does not move. He does not speak. If he does not soon, he will be given an electric shock, or two, or more. He will remain in 'involuntary custody' as long as he does not snap out of it one way or another. To authorize this procedure a psychiatrist (or two) signs a form, authorizing it to be done. As things are, how can it be otherwise?

If we wish some group to have the power to do to people whatever may be necessary to stop, start, or change them, there is no group in a better position to do so than psychiatrists. We should not blame psychiatrists because we give them such depth of power, especially when, to be exercised as expected, it *must* be exercised *routinely*.

One may be in hospital at one's own behest. Otherwise one is 'in' because the company one keeps does not find one congenial.

Not all psychiatric wards are 'locked', but everywhere in the developed world there is a psychiatric ward somewhere not too far away to which to send those who 'have to be locked up': for observation in the first place, then for a repertoire of possibilities, depending on the local psychiatric orientation – drugs, straitjackets, padded cells, tube feeds, injections, electroshocks, comas, lobotomies; maybe for behaviour therapy, or reconditioning of one kind or another.

All micro-social crises, the heartbreak and the catastrophes that so often lead to someone becoming a psychiatric patient in a mental institution, all go on outside these institutions. Even when a psychiatrist is called 'in' to such a situation, often he is expected to regard what he sees as a *fait accompli*; often he does, and it is. He gives his official seal, as it were, to the proceedings.

During my first six years of professional practice as a psychiatrist I hardly saw a patient outside institutions, whether mental hospitals, psychiatric units, out-patient clinics, or other wards or prisons. How many of these people got to those places in the first place was something of a mystery. What was going on *before* I, as a psychiatrist, appeared on the scene, whether on a 'home visit', or, much more usually, in my office or on the ward? One takes a 'history' from the patient, relatives, or friends to find out. I realized, often, that it would take something like a major detective investigation to find out. Working entirely 'in' institutions, I began to find it strange how people appeared in them, already metamorphosed into patients, voluntarily or involuntarily, self-'referred' or referred by a referring

doctor or social worker. Whence came they, out of that
world out there, where patients were people before they
were patients? And whither go they to become what or
whom again when they disappear? They are in-patients and
out-patients because of what they were like before they
were patients: whatever were they like when they were not
yet patients?

Mental hospitals and psychiatric units admit, routinely,
every day of the week, people who are sent 'in' for non-
criminal conduct, but for conduct which their nearest and
dearest relatives, friends, colleagues and neighbours find
insufferable. This is our society's only resolution to this
unlivable impasse. If they refuse to go away, or can't or
won't fend for themselves, it is our only way to keep people
out of the company that can't stand them. The staff of those
places to which such unpopular people are sent are paid
minimal wages to take care of them. It is not surprising that
the ordinary human beings who are the staff feel no more
need for such company than anyone else has done. Who
wants to get especially close to such rejected people who
end up as patients? Psychiatrists and nurses seldom have to
be reprimanded for getting too close to them and never for
not keeping a safe distance.

This state of affairs seems inevitable in those psychiatric
institutions that are prisons for people whom the world out
there can't stand and wants secluded and excluded for non-
criminal offences. To say that a locked ward functions as a
prison for non-criminal transgressors is not to say it should
not be so. Our society may continue to 'need' some such
prisons for unacceptable persons. As our society functions
at present such places are indispensable. This is not the
fault of psychiatrists, nor necessarily the fault of anyone.

Psychiatrists never tire of telling us that there is an un-
bridgeable gulf between some people and the rest of us. Karl
Jaspers called it an abyss of difference. Manfred Bleuler calls it
a total difference. No human bond can span it. Some people

are 'strange, puzzling, inconceivable, uncanny, incapable of empathy, sinister, frightening; it is impossible to approach them as equals', in Manfred Bleuler's words. Both he and Jaspers are talking about schizophrenics – over one in ten of us according to orthodox psychiatry.

These are extraordinary statements to have to be made, and not only on behalf of psychiatrists. They express feelings many people share. In the face of this, Harry Stack Sullivan, the American psychiatrist, felt impelled to announce that such people were, more than anything else, 'simply human'.

Carl Rogers tells me that Martin Buber told him once that schizophrenics are not capable of an I-Thou relationship. That sums up the psychiatric position, and that is the position from which I dissent. It is simply not a generalization I can make to match my own personal experience of such people. Psychiatrists say I am kidding myself, or that I am one of them anyway, or that I am trying to make out that these people do not need treatment. They do indeed 'need treatment'. Whatever treatment they get, first and last, 'we' should not forget to treat 'them', however strange 'they' are to 'us', as 'simply human' like ourselves.

There are many people who have been psychotic – in their own estimation as well as in that of psychiatrists – who want people to know what it is like to be completely out of the ordinary, commonsense, shared world, and into some other hell-world of sheer horror, terror and torture. There is no doubt that there are enormous differences between states of mind, between different 'realities'. I am not trying to gloss over or to minimize these differences. The question is: what sort of difference does this sort of difference make? What sort of difference does it make to 'us'? What sort of difference do we take the difference between us to be?

Without doubt there is loss of personal contact, lack of rapport, and so on. Why? Some psychoanalysts and psychotherapists strain to understand schizophrenese. There are schools which decode its signs and symptoms.

In some ways psychoanalytic systems of 'interpretation',

which try to make sense out of psychotic symptomatology, in making out that the patient means something totally different – if he or she means anything – from what he or she seems to mean, only widen the gulf. It is no surprise that there is no evidence that individual psychotherapy, based on such systems of proving to the patient that he or she is incapable of saying anything that in itself makes sense, seems to work.

Karl Jaspers maintained that there was 'no greater difference' in 'the psychic life' of human beings than that between the normal person and the psychotic. A corollary to this doctrine is that this difference is genetic and constitutional. It must be. This psychiatric doctrine of the abyss of difference between us and them takes us to the brink of another sort of abyss. How do 'we' treat 'them'? The Nazi regime in Germany in the late thirties took this doctrine to its logical conclusion. They should not be allowed to breed, and there was no point, really, in keeping them alive. They started their cleaning and tidying up of Germany by killing 50,000 mental-hospital patients until they stopped under protest from the Churches and others. But there was no general outcry against the theory and practice. They then switched the same exterminating teams over to the Jews and the gypsies.

A real Aryan Nazi would be psychotic to call himself a Jew. The Jewish parents of a lady schizophrenic patient of mine got out of Germany and settled in the Mid-West of the USA, where they passed themselves off as good German Lutherans. She was diagnosed schizophrenic when she began to have delusions that she was Jewish.

The attribution to the other of an incapacity to form a human bond was and is *the* basis for the diagnosis of schizophrenia. Both this attribution and the causal theory to account for it are crushed into the diagnosis. He or she is cut off (schizophrenic in a descriptive sense) and this is so *because* he or she is suffering from a mental illness, namely, schizophrenia, in the causal sense.

In my first book, *The Divided Self*, I tried to show the situation here. The attribution (the patient is autistic) is made by a person, in the role of diagnosing psychiatrist, about a person, in the role of patient-to-be-diagnosed. It is made across a gulf *between* them. The sense of a human bond with that patient may well be absent in the psychiatrist who diagnoses the patient as incapable of any such bond with anyone. Many psychiatrists have become very angry with me for pointing this out. Some enhanced understanding of what is going on between psychiatrist and patient does not preclude a scientific explanation of what is going on in the patient alone, and such a scientific explanation does not need to be a way to cut off a cut-off person from the possibility of human reunion, communion and renewal.

I have never idealized mental suffering, or romanticized despair, dissolution, torture or terror. I have never said that parents or families or society 'cause' mental illness, genetically or environmentally. I have never denied the existence of patterns of mind and conduct that are excruciating. I have never called myself an anti-psychiatrist, and have disclaimed the term from when first my friend and colleague, David Cooper, introduced it. However, I agree with the anti-psychiatric thesis that by and large psychiatry functions to exclude and repress those elements society wants excluded and repressed. If society requires such exclusion then exclusion it will get, with or without the aid of psychiatry. Many psychiatrists want psychiatry to bow out of this function. In Italy, as I have mentioned, some have done so; more would like to do so in other countries, but it is not easy. Such a complete change of policy requires as complete a change of outlook, and that is rare.

Thus society expects psychiatry to perform two very special functions. To lock certain people up; and to stop and, if possible, change certain states of mind and types of conduct in the name of curing mental illnesses.

Within two years of carrying out my duties as a clinical psychiatrist, I came to the painful realization that I would not like to be treated the way my own patients had to be treated. I would not like to be locked up in a psychiatric ward under observation. I could not believe that the drugs, the comas, the electric shocks I was expected to prescribe and administer were the great recent advances in psychiatry I was trained to believe they were. But maybe I had got it all wrong – I had to admit that if I were like many of my patients, there would be nothing else for it. The psychiatrists who were doing what I was supposed to learn to copy did not seem to be uncomfortable about what they were doing.

I knew what a psychiatrist like me was supposed to conclude about my patient's state of mind if he were to tell me my treatment was destroying him. But I agreed with him. Was I at the fuzzy beginnings of a clinical paranoid psychosis? Over thirty years later I am trying to put words to the unease I felt then and still feel about some aspects of the field of my profession.

There are hundreds of thousands of people in every country in the civilized world who lapse into wretched and crippling and crippled states of mind. If they get too much for us we turn them over to a psychiatric service they are not at liberty to refuse, and which is not at liberty to refuse them. Their wretched minds and rejected conduct now fall within the observation and control of psychiatry, which is given a twofold mandate. First, to keep such persons excluded from the ordinary outside world for as long as ordinary company out there cannot abide them. This can be and is done. The second mandate is to stop, if possible, to change, if possible, their conduct and states of mind from undesirable to desirable. These two duties are placed on psychiatry. It is ensured that psychiatrists carry out these tasks by giving them *power* to do so, a power *they* can't refuse, if they want to practise psychiatry.

There is a strange contradiction in society's attitude to psychiatric power. Psychiatrists are empowered by the law of the land. They do not ask for all that has been foisted on them. Some want more and some want less power in some respects. Some feel that psychiatry has been oversold. The hopes placed on it are unrealistic, the inevitable disillusion unpleasantly nasty. Yet, for all that, society demands that they exercise their power routinely, day in and day out. If all goes routinely, as it routinely does, they are not asked to answer to anyone but themselves. It is their job to make all the diagnoses they make. These diagnoses give the psychiatrist more power over the diagnosed than a judge has over a prisoner he condemns to prison. Yet, for all that power exercised routinely, and without a jury, when a psychiatrist makes the same diagnoses he usually makes routinely (which empower him to hospitalize a person and have him or her at his mercy) about a prisoner in the dock, before a judge and jury, prosecuting and defending counsel, his 'opinion' as often as not cuts no ice with them. Or, if it does, as often as not, it is in opposition to another psychiatric 'opinion', from an equally qualified psychiatrist, which cuts no ice. In courts of law psychiatric opinions are taken into serious consideration but by no means necessarily adopted. Yet, out of court, these same psychiatrists, with the same opinions, are invested with more power over persons whom only they say are to be patients or not than magistrates or judges over any accused. I was frightened by the power invested in me as a psychiatrist and by the way I was expected to use it.

Even more, I was frightened by the mind behind a lot of psychiatric theory and practice. I can best indicate what I mean by showing it in action.

Kierkegaard's *The Concept of Dread* is, by common acclaim, one of the most profound theological texts of the last 200 years. It was reviewed in the *American Journal of Psychiatry**
in 1944 by Abraham Myerson, a prominent psychiatrist from Boston. He wrote:

* Vol. 101, p. 839.

This book is interesting to the psychiatrist mainly because it inadvertently presents strong evidence that the writer is a psychiatric case himself and yet he has created quite an impression as a significant writer.

He offers us 'two representative samples of the style of the author' which 'adequately demonstrate that his book is a schizoid and certainly utterly incomprehensible presentation by a mind which is quite deviate'.

If sin is dealt with in psychology, the mood becomes persistence of observation, the dauntlessness of the spy, not the ardent flight of seriousness away from and out of sin . . . sin becomes a state. But sin is not a state. As a state (*de potentia*) it *is* not, whereas *de actu* or *in actu* it is and is again. The mood of psychology would be antipathetic curiosity, but the correct mood is the stouthearted opposition of seriousness.

And:

How sin came into the world every man understands by himself alone; if he would learn it from another, he *eo ipso* misunderstands it. The only science which can do a little is psychology, which nevertheless concedes that it does not, that it *can* and *will* not, explain more. If any science would explain it, everything would be brought to confusion. That the man of science ought to forget himself is perfectly true, but for this reason it is so fortunate that sin is not a scientific problem, and therefore the man of science is no more obliged than is any speculator to forget how sin came into the world. If he would do that, if he would magnanimously forget himself, he, with his zeal to explain humanity as a whole, becomes just as ridiculous as the privy counsellor who sacrificed himself to such a degree in leaving his visiting cards on Tom, Dick and Harry, that in doing so he finally forgot his own name.

These passages are as clear as crystal to me. I am in full accord with them. To a prominent representative of and spokesman for mainstream clinical psychiatry they speak for themselves. They are schizoid and certainly incomprehensible productions from a mind that is quite deviant. I realized with some dread that I was, from this psychiatric point of view, on the other and wrong side of that great divide that psychiatrists of this ilk are for ever telling us exists.

Such is how this sort of mind looks at life in theory. Myerson's practice is thoroughly consistent with his theory. Kierkegaard could easily be a patient just for being Kierkegaard, and be treated accordingly. In treatment, according to Myerson, 'there have to be organic changes or organic disturbances in the physiology of the brain for the cure to take place.' Disturbance in memory 'is probably an integral part of the recovery process.' There are some people who have 'more intelligence than they can handle' and a 'reduction in intelligence is an important factor in the curative process . . . some of the very best cures that one gets are in those individuals whom one reduces almost to amentia.'[1]

I cajoled one of my psychiatric superiors to read Kierkegaard's *The Sickness Unto Death*. He did. 'Thank you. Very interesting. A very good example of early nineteenth-century schizoid psychopathology,' he commented. At the same time, I dreaded much more than ever becoming like them and felt an enormous relief and sense of gratitude that I was not one of them. What was I to do, under these circumstances? Insofar as my mind was akin to Kierkegaard's, it suffered from the same psychopathology, schizoid, or worse. My mind went along also with such diagnosed psychotics as Nietzsche, Joyce, even *Artaud*! Worse! definitely. I had been trained to diagnose myself as schizophrenic.

Antonin Artaud:

You can say all you want about the mental health of
Van Gogh who, during his lifetime, cooked only one of

his hands, and other than that did no more than cut
off his left ear . . .

. . . present-day life goes on in its old atmosphere
of prurience, of anarchy, of disorder, of delirium, of
dementia, of chronic lunacy, of bourgeois inertia, of
psychic anomaly (for it isn't man but the world that
has become abnormal), of deliberate dishonesty and
downright hypocrisy, of a mean contempt for
anything that shows breeding,

of the claim of an entire order based on the
fulfilment of a primitive injustice,

in short, of organized crime.

Things are bad because the sick conscience now
has a vital interest in not getting over its sickness.

So a sick society invented psychiatry to defend itself
against the investigations of certain visionaries whose
faculties of divination disturbed it.[2]

This is psychosis. I had been trained to diagnose myself
psychotic.*

Anyone is at the risk, in almost any circumstances, as soon
as one is completely *at the mercy of other people*. If one is in
extreme mental confusion one is liable to be in extreme
jeopardy. I would not like to be at the mercy of this sort of

---

* On reading this passage in the typescript Dr Leon
Redler wrote me the following note:

When I was a psychiatric resident at Metropolitan
Hospital in New York City (1963–65) the consultant
on ward rounds used as a criterion for diagnosing a
man schizophrenic that he could not understand
what he was talking about. A fellow resident, now
on the faculty of the Harvard Psychiatry Dept.,
commented that he had real difficulty
understanding what Hegel was talking about. Would
the consultant, if he had similar difficulty and
indeed could not fathom Hegel, thereby diagnose
Hegel as schizophrenic? The consultant psychiatrist
replied: 'I certainly would.'

psychiatric mentality: nor at the mercy of other sorts of attitudes and practices that run through other divisions of medicine, not only psychiatry. I remember remarks made to me in all seriousness by psychiatrists. 'Hamlet was just a badly conditioned rat.' 'If Lear had been given electric shocks there would have been no need for all that nonsense.' Then again: a professor of psychiatry who heads a psychiatric unit in a general hospital (not in the UK) tells me that, if a psychiatrist is called in by another unit to sedate a noisy person, the service expected and provided is an injection and an electric shock from a bedside plug, in the ward, behind the usual screens. Surgeons can sedate people perfectly well themselves, but they call in the psychiatrist to 'press the button'. The patient comes round soon enough, effectively dazed and calm, unable, hopefully, to remember what he or she was going on about and mercifully disinclined to go on about anything. No 'permission' is asked of anyone. Neither the patient nor his or her relatives are told. Even other patients do not know. It may not be entered in the case notes.

This is not fair play. A psychiatrist admires Kierkegaard and Artaud. He sees no problem. What he does, pragmatically, routinely, frightens me. The fact that he sees no problem frightens me. The fact that he is merely acting as a cog in a much bigger wheel of routine, bland power frightens me. The fact that society hands people such power to exercise their own discretion on how to exercise the power they are given frightens me.

There is no more extreme dependence of one individual upon another in our society than at the interface between a psychiatrist examining someone psychiatrically and the person being examined. On the basis of possibly less than five minutes from the first laying on of eyes on a stranger, without that stranger perhaps ever having moved or said anything (so: he is either malingering, or he is a mute catatonic schizophrenic), a psychiatrist in any developed country can sign a printed form and make a phone call. This will be enough for that person to be taken away, imprisoned

and observed indefinitely. It may, and often does, inaugu-
rate a period of weeks, months or years during which that
person is kept imprisoned – that is, in involuntary custody –
and there drugged, regimented, reconditioned, brain given
electrical lavages, bits possibly taken out by knife or laser,
and anything else the psychiatrist decides to try out. This
autonomy given, indeed imposed on, psychiatry to strip
away civil rights and liberties in the name of the medical
necessity for observation and treatment has no equivalent in
any legally authorized power anywhere in our society, except, I suppose, where the torture of prisoners is legal.

It does not follow from such possibly disturbing considerations that the exercise of such power is not desirable
and necessary, or that, by and large, psychiatrists are not
the best people to exercise it, or, generally, that most of
what does happen in the circumstances is not the best that
can happen under the circumstances. I think it is a pity,
though, that almost everywhere it is all that *can* happen,
when, I often feel, it *needn't* be, if only . . .

Let us keep in focus the different functions a psychiatric
institution is expected to fulfil.

1. Voluntary and involuntary incarceration.

2. Stopping undesirable states of mind and forms of
   conduct.

3. Changing undesirable states of mind and forms of
   conduct into less undesirable or even desirable
   states of mind and conduct.

In every case, there is the question: undesirable to
whom? Often patients are as keen or keener to change as
anyone else is to change them. I think that most patients I
have encountered in psychiatric wards and clinics definitely
wanted, often desperately wanted, *help*. Then there is no
conflict. One offers them whatever one believes to be the
best help one can in the circumstances. The help one offers
will be entirely conditioned by what one believes the help

someone needs to be. Someone may appeal to one for help but the help one may believe that person to need could be the opposite of what he or she believes he or she needs. In which case? The help one psychiatrist thinks a patient needs may be the opposite of what other psychiatrists think. Psychiatrists often disagree; so do nurses; and psychiatrists, nurses, social workers, relatives and others all may disagree between themselves; any one person may be in two minds, and the patient may just want to be let out and let alone.

Most psychiatrists believe, for instance, that something should be done to the brain of someone who reports that their thoughts get blocked by external influences, that thoughts are stolen from and inserted into their minds by external agencies. Most psychiatrists believe that these experiences are due to some biochemical disorder in the central nervous system. Suppose the brain is like a TV set. The psychiatrist believes the interference is due to a disorder *in* the set. The patient believes the disorder in the programme is due to interference *to* the set. The analogy is not intended to validate its own validity. The key consideration is that the *way* we look determines *what* we see and what we think ought to be done, if anything.

Sometimes patients beg us to take away their thoughts. We do if we can. Sometimes patients beg us to let them keep their thoughts, and we take their thoughts away if we can, including the thought that they want to keep them. If treatment is successful they will be grateful to us that they cannot remember the thoughts we took away, and be grateful to us that we helped them not to want to keep them.

Euripides wrote: 'A slave is he who cannot speak his thoughts.' A patient may or may not be allowed to think them.

A medical institution is not the place to find freedom of thought and speech. I learned at school and at university to voice my thoughts and feelings with the greatest precaution and circumspection to teachers, tutors or professors. It is nerve-racking enough to be a medical student or young doctor under examination. How much *more* do such considerations apply when one is a *patient* and the *examination* is to pass or fail one's thoughts or feelings, brains, biochemistry, and to decide whether one is to be allowed to continue with them as they are.

Like Manfred Bleuler (whose father, Eugene Bleuler, coined the term 'schizophrenia'), I would like to believe that schizophrenia is 'a term of protection'. A mental hospital may still offer hospitality and sanctuary from what can happen outside. Nevertheless, the psychiatric 'treatment' of many people is still leaving behind it a trail of unsavoury things done in the name of treatment. If fear comes from the protector, who can protect us from fear? I am still more frightened by the fearless power in the eyes of my fellow psychiatrists than by the powerless fear in the eyes of their patients. I dread the thought of either look appearing in my eyes.

From a psychiatric point of view, the fact that many people are frightened to become patients of psychiatrists is not surprising. It only goes to show that there are many secret paranoid psychotics around, some of whom are paranoid about psychiatry and phobic about psychiatric treatment. Psychiatric treatment might destroy their delusions, one of them being that psychiatric treatment will destroy them.

Recently I asked a class of eighteen young psychiatrists from the Royal Bethlem Hospital in London what they would do if they decided I was psychotic but was not a danger to self or others, was not jeopardizing myself or family economically and did not want their treatment. Most of them felt that under the circumstances it would be their medical responsibility to 'treat' me if I 'needed' treatment, whether I thought I needed it or not. I can see exactly how they got to that position, but, I must admit – and I told them – it scares me.

The way we are taught to examine a patient psychiatrically, to elicit the signs and symptoms of the psychiatric condition, is an effective way to drive someone crazy, or more crazy. There is no camaraderie in this. Maybe if we could

learn to drive patients crazy, we could learn to drive them
sane – but how?

In any examination to become a qualified psychiatrist the
candidate is given a patient to 'examine', and then has to be
examined on the case by one of the examiners.

There are comparatively 'easy' cases and tricky or really
'nasty' cases. On first routine mental or physical examination, nothing abnormal may be detected (n.a.d.). Such a
patient who, to use the awful jargon, 'appears n.a.d.' may
well be one of those 'well-defended' paranoiacs who are too
paranoid to reveal their paranoid system to an examining
psychiatrist right away. But exams are there to be passed.

> He would not give away anything for the first twenty
> minutes, but I broke the bastard down, and out it all
> came, ideas of reference, thought control, the lot.

Exam candidates have to do what they have to do to pass
the examination. If one had 'let the patient get away with it',
one would have failed. In proper medical terminology, one
does not break the patient down: one elicits, like a neurologist, like any other doctor, the signs and symptoms of the
disease. One is sitting an examination in psychiatry to
establish that one is more skilful than a non-psychiatrically
trained doctor in doing so. Given such a patient, I would
have had to do the same, otherwise I would not be able to
write this now. Imagine having to *induce* cardiac failure in
order to pass an examination in cardiology. The last thing
one wants. We do not wish to induce cardiac decompensa-
tion when examining someone with cardiac incompetence.

> We don't hold much with talking to patients in this
> ward. Our main objective is to break the cycle of
> madness and get them out. *Charge Nurse, 1984*

Generally speaking, the type of psychiatrist I was trained to
be seldom sees anyone who is in a different state for longer
than it takes to decide whether to let it go on or to put a stop
to it. The detection of the existence of certain condemned

states of mind is sufficient reason to end them. The psychiatrist is condemned to know next to nothing of what he is putting a stop to.

Such was my job. It challenged me to think about this state of affairs. I could not share the assumption that all the conduct and experiences in question were so worthless and harmful that they should be stopped routinely. If one is always stopping them as soon as they rear their ugly heads, how can one know what would happen if one did not? I failed to develop the feeling that I had a *medical* mission to stop people, *against their will*, from feeling the way they did: the customary terms like archaic, alogical, irrational, primitive, palaeological, pathological, superstitious, savage, psychotic, seemed more a rhetoric of abuse than clinical descriptions.

I started off taking psychiatric theory and practice for granted. I never came to 'believe in' it and in the rhetoric used to describe and justify it. I began to wish I could jettison pretty well all of it. But what else could one do? No one likes the idea that, if one is in such extreme mental and emotional distress as to be helpless, one will be at the mercy of other people, including psychiatrists. What happens when they feel that things ought to be done *to* me which I do not feel ought to be done to anyone? No one knows what to do. What does one do, when one does not know what to do?

Both on humanitarian grounds and on scientific medical psychiatric grounds, I began to dream of trying out a whole new approach without exclusion, segregation, seclusion, observation, control, repression, regimentation, excommunication, invalidation, hospitalization (from the verb: to hospitalize) and so on: without those features of psychiatric practice that seem to belong to the sphere of social power and structure rather than to medical therapeutics. They might be 'therapeutic' but there is still no clinical, scientific, medical evidence of any kind that they are.

I wanted to clear a space where people, either defined as patients or not (that is a matter of *etiquette*), could be treated by me, if they wanted to be treated by me, in completely different ways, in many respects the *opposite* ways, from those in which I had been trained to treat them. Then we would see what happened. But, I was told, how can you? You are abdicating your medical responsibilities. It's like refusing to give a diabetic insulin. To encourage a schizophrenic to talk to you is like encouraging a haemophiliac to bleed. I knew that eventually I would have to have the courage of my lack of psychiatric convictions.

One young woman came to see me because she was beginning to feel a compelling longing or need not to move. If she became motionless, she could just about get herself moving again with great effort. Moreover, she felt an equally compelling pull within her to say nothing.

In other words she was moving into catatonic mutism for, as usual, no ascertainable reason.

I did not know what to suggest. She came to see me again several months later; she now felt able to move and talk perfectly well, though she had little inclination to do so more than was absolutely necessary.

She had got herself a job as a model in an art school. There she remained motionless and speechless for hours on end, and got paid for it. She had had the brilliant intuition to market her catatonia. Her job was the perfect therapy. She did not mind what position she was put in, as long as she could stay in it for a sizable length of time.

Her 'brain-wave', to get paid for doing just what she felt driven to do, would not work for everyone who could be given the same diagnosis. Most people who are drawn in her direction have other eccentricities that make life outside a psychiatric unit unfeasible for them, in our society. Nevertheless, it was suggested to me that the best strategy might not always be to try to stop the behaviour that is regarded as pathological. We have no idea why this sort of pull towards immobility overtakes some people.

That little old lady, tears streaming down her face, on her knees, wringing her hands, lips moving, no words uttered,

pleading. . . . There is no one there. Now she is listening.
There is no one there.

Is she an hallucinating psychotic in the locked ward of a
mental hospital? Is she saying her prayers in a cathedral?
She could be the same person.

A lady of thirty-eight comes to see me. In the last year she
has become beset by visual hallucinations which she wishes
to dispel. They are driving her frantic and she has become
reduced to going out of her house very seldom. She lives
with an older lady friend.

When she wakes up in the morning, the moment she
opens her eyes, before she can lift her head from the pillow,
a fist, the size of a man, is liable to crash through the ceiling
and stop just a hair's breadth from her eyes.

Penises rain down from the sky and sometimes sprout up
from the floor or from the ground.

If this lady were to consult almost any doctor in the
Western world, or any priest, she would almost certainly be
referred straight away to a psychiatrist. In her state of
agitation, hallucination and increasing isolation almost
every psychiatrist would recommend immediate admission
to a psychiatric unit for 'observation' and treatment. The
treatment would almost certainly be based on several
drugs, which she would be put on immediately, and after
adjusting the dosage, she would be discharged on the basis
of keeping on these drugs, maybe for years. There would be
a good chance that these drugs would inhibit her hallucinations a great deal; she would very likely feel less frantic and
agitated. She would almost certainly have to be on more
than one drug and almost certainly the dosages of all of
them would have to be high – not necessarily all that high in
comparative terms in psychiatric practice, but high in the
sense that if a normal person were suddenly to take in one
day what she would have to take every day, they would be
lucky if they were not rushed to hospital in deep coma. So
her system has to pay the price of having to adapt to such a

degree of chemicalization. All these drugs have effects on the system apart from the particular effect for which they are employed. These are called 'side-effects': simply, those effects the drug has that are not wanted.

However, there are thousands of patients who are very grateful to such medication and have no doubt that the price to pay – of unwanted effects – is well worth the result: inhibiting the mental activity that is occasioning them such distress.

As a clinical psychiatrist at Glasgow University, it fell to my lot to examine a patient referred to the psychiatric department from the ear, nose and throat department. The patient complained of deafness and intractable pain in his left ear, and after exhaustive examinations and investigations they could find nothing the matter with him.

I asked him what was giving him his pain in the ear. No one apparently had thought of asking him that question. If anyone had, no one *had* asked him. He told me. He was a dockyard worker and a Scottish Presbyterian, brought up in a way I know well. Every day as he walked to work and back from work he passed a fountain in a park topped by a statue of a naked lady. As he passed the statue he could feel his eyeballs moving in the direction of the naked lady, though he kept his neck from turning round. As his eyes turned round, however, he got a sharp kick in his earhole from his guardian angel. He knew she was about three feet tall, robed in white, and hovered above and behind his left shoulder. He had never dared to try to look at her.

We are plunged into a world far different from the world of ordinary medicine.

He often felt cold. When he was cold he felt frightened and guilty. He did not know why. But he discovered, if he warmed himself standing with his back to a coal fire, that as he felt warmer he felt less frightened of being eaten by himself, and at the same time less guilty. Is it not remarkable that a change of temperature changed so much else, far more quickly and completely than any of the many drugs he had taken to allay his fears?

As his body warmed up, he could return to his old self, remember things he had forgotten, make plans for the future, forget frantic anxieties he had been tortured by a few minutes before, feel good, physically and morally, regain a sense of humour, work out problems in mathematics (which he could not address himself to when cold), feel love again for his wife and children. But he had to heat himself in this special way, and after a while he had to roast himself to retain an effect that, when he had first hit on this device, had come with quite gentle warming.

A lecturer in sociology told me this story out of sociological interest.

At the end of one summer he felt 'a bit wobbly' just before the academic term was due to start. He went to his GP for some pills, and was recommended a rest in hospital for a weekend. He went in for a weekend, left after seventy-two hours, somewhat rested, and went back to work as usual. That was that. Nine years later he applied for the renewal of his driving licence. It was renewed and has been renewed again, but now only on a short-term basis. When he enquired into the reason for this he received a letter explaining that nine years ago when in hospital for a rest he had been diagnosed as having a 'bipolar affective disorder', a 'recurrent' condition.

And so, although it had not recurred, he was now suffering from '*a prospective mental illness*'.

> Psychopharmacological drugs
> which are claimed to be active in the clinic,
> whether anti-depressant like imipramine,
> or antipsychotic or neuroleptic,
> like reserpine or chlorpromazine,
> have a very marked anti-mescaline activity
>
> in the mouse.*

* James Fenton, from 'Exempla', *The Memory of War*, Penguin, 1983, p. 75.

Drugs can be a great boon in psychiatry or any other style of mental healing. It all depends on how they are used or abused.

There are drugs to calm agitation, to soften frantic feelings, to tone down awful moods, to modulate the tonal region of feelings, to regulate thoughts and the style and content of imagination and dreams. If no one and nothing can bring one out of suicidal depression, there are electric shocks. They may abolish insufferable thoughts and feelings, at least for a while, maybe forever. If I were being driven frantic by mental and emotional torment that nothing I or anyone or any drug could stop I might beg for electric shocks. Other people might beg to have electric shocks. The critical issue is the politics of the matter. Who has the power to do what to whom against whose will?

I lost any sense of desire or duty to force on people treatment that I would not want forced on me. Whatever else it has to do with, the issue has to do with human relationships.

Martin Buber laments what he calls the 'decrease in man's power to relate . . . he has divided his life with his fellow men into two neatly defined districts: institutions and feelings, It-district and I-district.' Institutions are 'out there' where 'one spends time, where one works, negotiates, influences, undertakes, competes, organizes, administers, officiates . . .'[3]

Institutions and feelings are not necessarily two 'neatly defined' districts. When I lived in hospitals I found a great deal of human warmth and camaraderie in them.

Institutions, for Buber, are 'out there'. During my first years as a doctor they were not 'out there' for me. They were the air I breathed. 'Out there' was the world, from which patients came. My fellow doctors and nurses went out there in off-duty hours. Without our uniforms or white coats we went to concerts, dances, theatres, cinemas, restaurants, pubs; we visited friends, relatives and maybe lovers who lived out there. We had to be careful not to

become institutionalized, however, to make a point of
keeping up 'outside contacts', to go to parties where one
could mingle with 'lay' people. It is easy to get out of
contact with that world outside just because one could find
more companionship inside. Such companionship tends to
develop between members of staff or between patients;
seldom between staff and patients. Even this is not a
universal generalization.

It can become economically and otherwise embarrassing
when patients start to regard the institution as their home,
to feel more at home inside than in the cold, bleak world
out there. People out there do not 'understand', and it is
impossible to explain. For myself, as a member of staff,
even when I had married and had a child, I remained very
drawn towards staying 'in' for as long as possible. A
hospital can be a good womb or a bad womb. It is a totally
different experience according to whether one *can* leave or
not. In Gartnavel, we reduced all drugs to virtually zero in
one locked ward and in the first week about thirty windows
were smashed. No one was hurt. We unlocked the door.
The windows stopped being smashed. There was no rush
to leave. As soon as people could leave, hardly anyone
wanted to.

Staff and patients can both be on the same side and on
the 'right side' of each other. Efforts in this direction within
psychiatry are not necessarily doomed. 'Power-sharing',
sharing 'responsibility' for 'decisions', are shibboleths of
the therapeutic-community movement within institutional
psychiatry. But it is difficult, as every professional who
has tried it knows very well, really to share power with
patients. Even when the staff would like to, sometimes,
in some respects. The power invested in the staff by
law does not include the power to give it away. That
would 'to abdicate one's medical responsibilities'. What
one does not allow, one forbids. What one does not
forbid, one allows. One is not allowed not to forbid what
one is forbidden to allow. Psychiatrists are themselves

constrained, not only for therapeutic reasons, to constrain patients in hospital wards.

Sleeping and waking, eating, drinking, digesting, urinating, defecating and breathing are biological basics. These basics are deeply socially programmed. They are all subject to disturbance. A great deal of the disturbances doctors are asked to treat are socially conditioned disturbances of these socially conditioned, biological, organic functions.

They are conditioned by injunctions made effective in many more ways than straight commands and prohibitions, rewards and punishments and more subtle quasi-hypnotic procedures. One need not be told to go to bed. One need not be told to be tired. One is told one *is* tired. Later one is tired when one was told one will be, without having to be told any more. We put ourselves to bed. We sleep then, not before. We sleep for a set length of time, not too little, not too much, wake up, get out of bed, and go through the day.

We eat not too much, nor too little, not loudly, not too fast, nor too slowly, not with all fingers at once. Any socially conditioned function can become deconditioned.

From a purely therapeutic point of view, it might not always be the best thing to clamp down on a deconditioned function with drugs and regimentation. But the structure of the usual psychiatric ward and the way a ward 'has to be run' make the possibility of letting people find and have their own rhythm out of the question. In a free society everyone's rhythm and tempo is free, as long as we do not transgress on others.

The principle of *autorhythmia* entails that each person has his or her own biorhythm and a right to this rhythm, and no person has a right to interfere with the rhythm and tempo of anyone else if it is not doing anyone harm. I would welcome intervention from others whether I liked it or not if I went into some of the hypermanic states I've seen in which I would die of exhaustion if I were not stopped.

This is in marked contrast to any regime, whether

monastic, regimental or psychiatric, voluntary or involuntary, where once within it one can come and go only in so far as one is allowed to – go to bed, sleep, get up, wake, wash, eat; the same thing, at the same time.

'Can I help you?' says the patient in a locked back ward to the nurse, who is carrying a pile of laundry to take along to the laundry room.

'I know what you're after. You just stay where you are. You've been out enough today,' snaps the nurse, as she unlocks the door with her key and slams it behind her.

Staff are 'institutionalized' along with the patients.

I could see the necessity for regimentation and routine, the way rules and roles have to be to make the system work. But I began to question the necessity of that sort of regime.

In hospitals and in mental hospitals and in-patient psychiatric units where biorhythm is under surveillance, and control, this power of control over the biorhythm of patients usually takes the form of regimentation. That is, it has to do with doing things at the same time; the 'ward' has to be in bed, silent, asleep, up, eat the same food, at the same time. A lot of medication is required to keep up this regimentation. Patients have to be drugged to sleep, and drugged to keep awake.

To allow 'day-night reversal' can very seldom be considered a practical possibility within psychiatric wards. Regimentation of biorhythm is an integral component in the efficient running of any hospital, psychiatric or otherwise. A hospital is not the place to be if one is into being up all night and asleep all day.

This is a difficult thought to take further in hospital. A hospital cannot run on autorhythmia for staff or patients any more than railways and airports for staff or passengers. In that case, maybe hospitals are not the best sort of place for some of the people who are in them.

It depends on how one looks at it. There is nothing intrinsically pathological about being awake at night and sleepy during the day. Most of my reading, thinking, writing has happened at night. Solitude, silence, desolation, camaraderie, romance, meditation, prayer, vigil, carousing, music, the moon, the stars, the dawn: there is no possibility of any of that sort of thing in almost any psychiatric unit. Maybe some people need the night. Where in the world are lunatics allowed to bathe naked in the moonlight?

Many people want the regimes we have. I am not arguing against them, so much as wondering what it would be like if it were all different: seen in a different way.

As a patient, other people decide with whom and how I spend my time. What positions I am to adopt (lying down, squatting, sitting, walking, standing, moving or motionless), when, where, in what company. What sounds are appropriate, when, where, with whom. How I dress. When, where, with whom, together or alone, how long I sleep and am awake. When, where, what, with whom I eat. I am stripped of almost all discretion and responsibility for every single observable detail of my life. What would happen, I began to wonder, if we were to declare *epistemological experiential anarchy*, and let everyone have their own biorhythm (*the principle of autorhythmia*) on the one hand, but on the other restrict or ban *transgressive conduct*, whatever anyone's real or presumed state of mind, motives or intentions?

We should be careful not to allow one sort of psychiatric sensibility to acquire a monopoly of power to stamp its mentality on us. One in four of all 'beds' (as the jargon goes) in all hospitals in the USA is 'occupied' by a schizophrenic. Roughly speaking there is about ten times more chance of being admitted to a mental hospital in any First World country than of being admitted to a university.

Whatever else is disturbing about what is going on on the surface of our planet, we can all agree that relations between human beings, industrial, economic, international, racial, sexual relations, and between so-called sane and so-called insane, are riven by distrust and strife. Camaraderie crops up as a sort of hobby, possibly a need, an addiction, like sex or golf or heroin. It would be surprising if it cropped up often between psychiatric staff and patients when there has to be, for the present system to work, such a vast difference of power between them. You can't let patients get away with it or they'll think they can get away with it. Don't get caught in collusions by false sentimentality. If you give them an inch they'll take a mile. Keep your distance. Keep them in their place. Don't lose yourself in 'over-identifying' with them. Don't inflame the psychotic process by rewarding psychotic symptomatology. It goes without saying that sexual intimacy between patients and between staff and patients is forbidden.

Even the institutionalized parody of normal communication is institutionally excommunicated. Thereafter, and possibly, I suggest, maybe also *therefore*, 'it' 'deteriorates': an aberration of normality 'deteriorates' into an aberration of an aberration. This secondary 'deterioration' seems to be necessarily an almost necessary, an almost inevitable development, given what mental hospitals seem to continue to have to be.

Can a psychiatric institution exist for 'really' psychotic people where there is communication within *solidarity*, community and communion, instead of the It-district, the no-man's-land between staff and patients?

This rift or rent in solidarity may be healed *in* a professional therapeutic relationship. A 'relationship', professional or otherwise, which does not heal this rent can hardly be called therapeutic since it seems to me that what is professionally called a 'therapeutic relationship' cannot exist without a primary human camaraderie being present and manifest. If it is not there to start with, therapy will have been successful if it is there before it ends.

There can be no solidarity if a basic, primary, fellow human feeling of being together has been lost or is absent.

It is not easy to retain this feeling when you press the button. Very seldom, when I pressed the button, could I feel I was doing for this chap in terrible mental agony what I hoped he would do for me if I had his mind and brains and he had mine.

This issue of solidarity and camaraderie between me as a doctor and those patients did not arise for me, it did not occur to me until I was in the British Army, a psychiatrist and a lieutenant, sitting in padded cells in my own ward with completely psychotic patients, doomed to deep insulin and electric shocks in the middle of the night. For the first time it dawned on me that it was almost impossible for a patient to be a pal or for a patient to have a snowball's chance in hell of finding a comrade in me.

It would be a mistake to suppose that 'mental' institutions are It-districts. There may be a lot of camaraderie between staff and staff, and patients and patients. But there tends to be an It-district between staff and patients. Why this should be so may not be immediately apparent. But when one looks into it one sees that it can hardly be otherwise, under the circumstances.

All communication occurs on the basis either of strife, camaraderie or confusion. There can be communication without communion. This is the norm. There is very little communion in many human transactions. The greatest danger facing us, the human species, is ourselves. We are not at peace with one another. We are at strife, not in communion.

The New Year is the biggest celebration in Scotland. It is marked by prolonged carousing on the part of the alcoholic fraternity, but many teetotallers celebrate the spirit of the New Year contentedly sober. There is no 'religion' about it. There is a special spirit abroad – 'Auld Lang Syne', 'A man's a man for a' that.' In Gartnavel, in the so-called 'back wards', I have seen catatonic patients who hardly make a move, or utter a word, or seem to notice or care about anyone or anything around them year in and year out, smile, laugh, shake hands, wish someone 'A guid New Year' and even dance . . . and then by the afternoon or evening or next morning revert to their listless apathy. The change, however fleeting, in some of the most chronically withdrawn, 'backward' patients is amazing. If any drug had this effect, for a few hours, even minutes, it would be world famous, and would deserve to be celebrated as much as the Scottish New Year. The intoxicant here however is not a drug, not even alcoholic spirits, but the celebration of a spirit of fellowship.

There are interfaces in the socio-economic–political structure of our society where communion is impossible or almost impossible. We are ranged on opposite sides. We are enemies, we are against each other before we meet. We are so far apart as not to recognize the other even as a human being or, if we do, only as one to be abolished immediately.

This rift or rent occurs between master and slave, the wealthy and the poor, on the basis of such differences as class, race, sex, age.

It crops up also across the sane-mad line. It occurred to me that it might be a relevant factor in some of the misery and disorder of certain psychotic processes; even sometimes, possibly, a salient factor in aetiology, care, treatment, recovery or deterioration.

This rift or rent is healed through a relationship with anybody, but it has to be somebody. Any 'relationship' through which this fracture heals is 'therapeutic', whether it is what is called, professionally, a 'therapeutic relationship' or not. The loss of a sense of human solidarity and camaraderie and communion affects people in different ways. Some people never seem to miss it. Others can't get on without it. It was not easy to retain this feeling when I pressed the button to give someone an electric shock if I could not feel I was doing to him what I hoped he would do for me if I had his brains and he mine. I gave up 'pressing the button'.

TWO

Family and School

FAMILY

The story of my 'background', from my father and mother, grandfather, father's grandfather's sister, mother's mother, aunts and uncles, true or false, was passed on to me as fact.

My father's family counted themselves as Vikings who had settled in north-east Scotland. They came from further north than north-east Scotland. They came from further north and east, from where they had forgotten – Scandinavia, probably Norway. My mother's family counted themselves Celtic Protestants from the south-west of Scotland.

On my father's side everyone had blue eyes, on my mother's side they all had dark eyes. I have dark eyes. I often thought my mother looked almost Spanish, almost Jewish.

On my father's side there was a great-aunt who taught classics. A great-uncle of my father's held the record as the oldest student to graduate at Aberdeen University and obtained his MA when he was seventy-five. Among my relatives on both sides of the family, the occupations were ceramics, painting on glass and china, schoolteachers, crofters, ministers of religion. My father's father was a naval architect. My father was apprenticed in a shipyard, Mavers and Colston, on the Clyde when he was fourteen, joined the Royal Tank Corps as a private when he was seventeen and ended the war as a lieutenant in the Royal Air Corps, and spent the rest of his working life as an electrical engineer in the service of the Corporation of

Glasgow, specializing in the maintenance of the electrical power and mains supply to the City of Glasgow.

He was also, for over twenty years, principal baritone in Glasgow University Chapel Choir. In this capacity he met many distinguished visiting musicians. I think his greatest pleasure in that respect was singing with Albert Schweitzer as organist and afterwards going out for a walk with him. His greatest hero, of his and my own time, was Mahatma Gandhi.

My paternal grandmother claimed, on her side of the family, Robert Louis Stevenson as a great-uncle, and hence George Stevenson, R. L.'s father, as a forebear. R. L. Stevenson is still best known in some parts of the highlands and islands of the west of Scotland as the son of George Stevenson, the builder of lighthouses in those parts. One of my earliest memories is of being taken to one of his light-houses in the Firth of Clyde. I was scolded for touching some vast sheet of glass. But it may all have been a dream.

Celts or Vikings, on both sides they were Scottish for several hundred years back. The only known other blood in the family did not run through my veins. One of my mother's sisters had married an Englishman. He was treated perfectly civilly.

My grandparents lived through the Boer War. My parents and all adults had lived through the Great War. I lived through the end of gaslit streets and horses and carts, the Spanish Civil War, and World War II. I was born the year after the General Strike of 1926 when tanks were out in the streets of Glasgow on Winston Churchill's orders. The Great War, the Last War, was supposed to have been the *last* war, the war to end all wars. There was a League of Nations. But no one I knew believed that fairy tale. No one was surprised, as we all listened to Chamberlain on the radio telling us that after some delay the curtain had gone up at last. No one at all in my whole environment, my mother, father, grandfather, aunts, uncles, schoolteachers, other children, family friends, believed that there was not going to be another war, a terrible war, more terrible than ever before.

When World War II started no one could imagine how it could possibly end without endless devastation, poison gas, germ warfare, torture, mutilation, rape, pillage, massacres, killing and killing and killing, shelling, bombing, sea warfare, food shortage, famine and pestilence, and not for the first and probably not the last time in history. But we all thought (there was only this one thought) this must be the end of civilization as we knew it. Not, as we now surmise, the end of the whole macro-biosphere and ecosystem.

H. G. Wells's vision in *The Shape of Things to Come* and *Mind at the End of its Tether* did not seem the least unlikely to the working and middle classes of my neck of the woods on the south side of the Clyde. Jews, Christians (Catholic and Protestant), atheists, religious nihilists, Labour or Tory, Communists said, 'Yes, the World Revolution is inevitable; there will be many, many deaths, but you cannot make an omelette without breaking a few eggs.' Willie Gallacher, Glasgow's Communist MP, was fond of reminding us of this on his soap-box on Sunday nights. This was it. We were in for it now. Gas masks reminded us. We all went to school with our gas masks. We might have to use them *anytime*. Air-raid shelters, air-raids. A gem of a Greek Thomson Church just up the road, up Dixon Road, near Queen's Park, in rubble the next morning.

Hiroshima, Nagasaki, the concentration camp documentaries. I had, no one had, ever seen anything like those first shots of Belsen, Buchenwald, Auschwitz, as the Americans and British moved in. I was stunned. Was that *it*? Or were there more horrors yet to come?

When the war finally ended there was enormous relief. Bonfires in the streets through the night, singing, dancing, carousing, crowds, all arm in arm, and as far as I can remember no hooliganism, no violence.

Yet no one I knew, as far as I can remember, believed

that *this*, the end of the war, was going to be the end of destruction and slaughter. It could not stop at Hiroshima and Nagasaki. This could only be the beginning of things to come. This was only a pause, but thank God for that.

The atmosphere then was quite unlike the periodic nuclear scares and crises of the subsequent thirty-six years. We knew we were doomed – unless a miracle happened. Quite a few people believed in miracles and millions prayed that by the Grace of God alone, through a miracle, the hearts of men might relent, forgive, repent, and all might lay down arms, and stop being nasty to each other and realize our brotherhood and sisterhood before God in a life of enjoyment, celebration and beatitude. Like almost everyone else, I believed that something like another war, or worse, had to happen. It was as though we were on a crash course on a train, trying to stop it by jumping at the rear walls of our carriage. We had already fallen from the Empire State Building and had only a few more feet before impact.

Short of a miracle, we could not imagine that we were not just about to bring our civilization to an end.

BEING GOOD

The system of punishment I was brought up with was relatively benign and straightforward. I was punished (i) for disobedience, (ii) for *what* I did wrong – that is, both for disobedience, which is wrong in itself, and for what, in being disobedient, I had done which I should not have done, because it was wrong in itself to do that, whether I had been told to or not. I was told not to do things only because it was wrong for me to do them.

I was taught not to pick my nose; not to slouch in a chair; not to put a finger in my ear; not, of course, to put a finger in my mouth; not to keep my mouth open; not to hum and haw; not to make a noise when eating; not to drink out of a saucer, let alone to slop anything on it in the first place; to lift a teacup up to my lips, not my lips down to it, with two fingers; to blow my nose properly; how to brush my teeth, comb my hair, tie my shoe laces, do my tie, always to have my socks pulled; how to shit properly and wipe my arse properly; not to turn up my eyes; how to speak properly; when and to whom to speak, with proper diction – for instance not 'sing-song' or some of the at least half-dozen forbidden accents, and a considerable amount of vulgar vocabulary.

From the age of seven I was expected to get myself up in the morning, do my teeth, wash my hands, arms, face, neck, gargle, pee and do No. 1, wash, wipe and dry my hands and all parts, put on my clothes correctly, brush my hair, sit down for breakfast on time, eat it not reading a book, check myself in the mirror, put on cap and, if necessary, galoshes, scarf, coat, gloves, and with a kiss and 'cheerio' be off to school with fare there and back, a clean handkerchief, a pen, a pencil, a ruler, a rubber, a geometry set, a pocket knife, and my books in my bag on my back.

I would be back at four-thirty unless it was an afternoon at the playing field, when it would be later. Then out for a music lesson or out to play. Back by six for tea when my father would have come home, practise before it was too late for the neighbours, maybe a bit of radio, 'The Brains Trust' (C. E. M. Joad, Julian Huxley, the anonymous Scottish doctor whom I later discovered to have been Edward Glover, the psychoanalyst), 'Henry Hall's Guest Night', Charlie Kunz and Chopin; and then homework, and then bath, bed, prayers and sleep, or the fire, bed, prayers and sleep, negotiated through a reverse process from the morning of undressing, bathing, peeing, doing No. 1, washing my hands and then to bed, lights out, no reading, no talking.

For most of the time (except for one or two incidents which I shall describe), apart from when there were minor frictions, provided I looked all right, smelt all right and sounded all right, as long as my thoughts were good and my heart was pure, I was as free as a bird.

If I had done my practice and my homework and if it was not my bedtime I was perfectly entitled to sit musing in front of the fire. Neither my mother nor my father would see any reason to interrupt me without some special reason. We lived a quiet life. There were hardly ever any special reasons. The same with practising, homework, reading. I was never unfairly interrupted.

I would lie in bed in any position I wanted. Provided I kept quiet, I did not have to be asleep.

As long as you do this (and that's not asking too much considering what we have done and are doing and will still have to do for you) and don't do that (and there is a good reason for our telling you everything we tell you not to do), you need feel no guilt or shame for anything you think, feel, imagine or do, provided it is not bad.

You *know*, we don't have to tell you, when you are doing wrong. You *know* if you are telling a lie. You *know* (you are not depraved) what is a clean thought and a dirty thought. You *know*, we don't have to tell you, the difference between the truth and a lie and when you are telling the truth and when you are lying. And you *know*, we don't have to tell you, how to respect yourself (i.e. not masturbate), and how to respect the other sex. If you are in any doubt, remember that *God* sees it all, everything, all the time. Let your mind and your heart, your words and your deeds be, as they are anyway (that's the funny thing, isn't it?), an open book to God.

When I was five, shortly before I was six, I was subject to running eczema. It took the form of many water blisters, which became easily infected, usually with a reddened area around them, which sprouted on my arms and lower legs, never on my head, face, neck or trunk.

My mother was 'very particular' about food. Rusks or toast. Honey, treacle, butter. No margarine, sweets, 'cheap' jam, Coca-Cola or anything like that.

When I went to school my mother reminded me of the dangers of putting anything into my mouth given me by anyone and made me make a solemn promise that I would not eat in particular any jam, margarine, rolls, bread or anything remotely like jam.

On my first day at school during the lunch-break a boy offered me, in exchange for one of my rusks, a bite of his large, very white roll with a thick layer of probably margarine and bright red jam in the middle. One had to open one's mouth to its widest to encompass it for a bite: I had a fair-sized bite. It all tasted delicious. The jam had a real cheeky taste, quite unlike honey.

That was my first taste of that trashy jam that rots everyone's teeth and would ruin my mother in spending a fortune on ointments, cotton wool, white lint and pink lint and green waterproofing and bandages, one-inch and half-an-inch, if ever any of that poison got into my system.

When I came home my mother made me look her in the eye and tell her the truth. Did I eat anything I had promised not to today at school?

No.

Is that the truth?

Yes.

Are you sure?

Yes.

You've lied to me, Ronald, and I'm going to tell your father when he comes home. And he'll give you a thrashing for breaking your promise to me and for lying to me.

And that was that. When my father came home my mother told him and he gave me a 'sound' thrashing, one degree severer than a 'good' thrashing.

Before I said my prayers that night I had to promise never to lie to my mother or father in future and never to eat any of those things I knew very well not to and which were *bad* for me and had promised once and broken my promise and now was promising again *never* to eat.

In the next three months I kept my promise. But after a few weeks I did come out in eczema as never before and, despite it costing my mother a fortune, it remained chronic, with only occasional short-lived intermissions, for the next three years.

My mother asked me a number of times in those three months, as she had done before, whether I had eaten anything. I replied truthfully that I had not and my mother believed me.

After three months my forearms, wrists and hands were almost always swathed in bandages through which the fluid from the water blisters would ooze to the outside.

I did not know why this was happening to me and everyone else was equally puzzled, at a loss. After about two months the rash evaporated.

I did not think that the mouthful of that 'jelly piece' Charlie had given me months ago could do this to me now and I had already been punished, I thought, for breaking my promise and lying, so it couldn't be that. In particular, I got this eczema without eating sweets, or other forbidden things. Then, after a while, it went away and I've been clear of a rash for months. Since I've got it *anyway*, why not accept that jelly baby, put it between my teeth, run my tongue around the portion of the jelly baby on the inside of my teeth, then pick it out of my mouth deftly and throw it away when no one is looking? This way it could not be said to have entered my mouth, I would not have bitten it, my lips would not have touched it, none of it would have come into contact with more than two fingers, two teeth, and the tip of my tongue.

I put this plan into operation with a jelly baby one Saturday at the corner of Victoria Road and Calder Street.

When I came in for lunch my mother asked me whether I had still kept my promise. She cautioned me carefully and I reiterated more than three times that I was telling the truth.

She then said that when she had been out shopping just before one o'clock the mother of one of my playmates had met her casually on the street and told her that her son had told her that I had eaten a jelly baby that he had given me and she was surprised because she thought I wasn't allowed to eat sweeties because they brought me out in that terrible rash.

I denied that I had eaten any jelly baby or had *taken* any jelly baby from him. There the matter remained until about two o'clock when there was a ring at the door and there was the boy who had given me the jelly baby asking Mummy if Ronald could come out to play. He had never come round to the house before.

My mother asked him in for a moment. He came into the sitting room.

'Did you give Ronald a jelly baby this morning?' not in the least ominously.

'Yes,' he said.

'No, you didn't!' I exclaimed.

But it was too late. He hadn't twigged it in time and he might have been a 'clipe' (informer) anyway.

We both of us had to stick to our story. Our three other companions of the morning were just out in the street waiting for us to go out to play. My mother *and* father called them up. Two of them couldn't remember, one thought he could, yes, I had taken a jelly baby – why, couldn't I remember? – when we had come out of the sweetie shop in Victoria Road just round the corner from Calder Street?

That was it. I admitted I had *taken* a jelly baby, I had held it in two fingers, put it between two front upper and lower teeth (which teeth? I was asked, and I showed her) and without it touching anything else I had licked the inside less than half of it with my tongue, briefly, and spat it out.

The boys were dismissed. They were told I wouldn't be going out to play with them now, and after a brief sentence was formally passed, I was given a really good, sound thrashing by my father on the floor, while my mother stayed out of the room.

Not long after going to school, Dad, Mummy and I were having dinner.

'This cabbage tastes like a lead pencil,' I voiced aloud, off my guard for a moment.

In a flash my mother exclaimed, 'How do you know what a lead pencil tastes like?' and, with a glance at my father, I was down on the floor for another memorable thrashing.

One of my consoling thoughts as I was being thrashed was, 'I'm never going to forget this.'

After that I don't think my mother ever trusted me, and I became very wary of her.

My mother could be a very tricky person.

In *Self and Others* I wrote up anonymously the story of one of her 'wiles' – the last one, I hoped, I would ever be caught in.

A boy of seven had been accused by his father of having stolen his pen. He vigorously protested his innocence but was not believed. Possibly to save him from being doubly punished as a thief and a liar, his mother told his father that he had confessed to her that he had stolen the pen. However, the boy still would not admit to the theft, and his father gave him a thrashing for stealing and for lying twice over. As both his parents treated him as though he both had done the deed and had confessed it, he began to think that he could remember having actually done it after all, and was not even sure whether or not he had in fact confessed. His mother later discovered that he had not in fact stolen the pen, and admitted this to the boy, without however telling his father. She said to the boy:

'Come and kiss your mummy and make it up.'

He felt in some way that to go and kiss his mother and make it up with her in the circumstances was somehow twisted. Yet the longing to go to her, embrace her, and be at one with her again was so strong as to be almost unendurable.

Although he could not articulate the situation clearly, he stood his ground without moving towards her. She then said: 'Well, if you don't love your mummy I'll just have to go away,' and walked out of the room.

The room seemed to spin. The longing was

unbearable but suddenly, everything was different yet
the same. He saw the room and himself for the first
time. The longing to cling had gone. He had
somehow broken into a new region. He was alone.
Could this woman be connected to him? As a man he
thought this incident crucial in his life: a deliverance,
but not without a price to pay.*

SANTA CLAUS

Like all the children I knew, and millions of others, I was
told that Santa Claus came down the chimney with the toys
on my bed and in my Christmas stocking on Christmas
morning. Apart from Santa Claus other people gave me
presents at Christmas – Mummy and Daddy, Grannie,
Auntie Ethel, even Old Pa and Auntie Maisie. I did not
know why, but I had no objections.

I believed in Santa Claus. Then came the Christmas after
my fifth birthday. I had had one term at school. It was not
that I disbelieved in him but I couldn't understand how he
could get down and up such a narrow chimney, no soot,
and down and up so many hundreds and hundreds of
chimneys in one night. However, Christmas was the birthday of Jesus, God's son and God incarnate. God could do
anything. But how? At school, some children said they
knew but were not telling.

I kept asking my parents. They said nothing. I tried to
stay awake all night to catch him. But I fell asleep and woke
up to find those maddening presents from Santa Claus
there again.

My mother later told me it had taken her about an hour
to crawl on the floor to my bed and back, because I kept on
'making starts'.

'*How* did Santa Claus get those presents there?' At
breakfast I was almost frantic. My parents gave me time
to guess. I couldn't.

* Penguin, 1960, pp. 163–4.

'*Think*,' they said, 'and we won't have to tell you. *Who* is Santa Claus?'

I gave up. '*Who* is Santa Claus?'

'*We* are!'

'*You are!?*' It had never occurred to me.

I knew my mother and father were sitting looking at me, waiting for me to thank them for all these lovely presents. I couldn't. I was stunned. Pain grabbed my throat. Santa Claus was *them*. I hated Santa Claus and them for being the same. I felt sorry for them, I could not be grateful. I thanked them. The toys did not interest me.

Millions of children 'find out' about Santa Claus without being upset at all. But I was physically panic-stricken. Why? It was an extreme intellectual crisis in a five-year-old. Santa Claus came down the chimney and left toys. How? No, not how does, but who is Santa Claus? Who is God? If they could be Santa Claus, God above knows what else they might not be.

This incident made me wary of believing anything because I was told it. I believed in God and Jesus maybe less than I believed in Santa Claus. I believed they existed because I was told they existed. I believed what I was told. It never occurred to me not to till then.

Toys came from Santa Claus because my parents told me they did. Toys came from Santa Claus, and Santa Claus was Santa Claus whoever he was. If Santa Claus was not Santa Claus, there was no Santa Claus. They told me they were Santa Claus. If they were Santa Claus, there was no Santa Claus. If they were God, there was no God.

Next Christmas I smashed the toys they gave me.

SCHOOL

Cuthbertson's Street School was the local council primary school.

Before going to school, I don't remember playing with any children. Playing with children of my age was synonymous with what we as adults rather awkwardly try to say when we use an expression like 'having a relationship' with children of my age. As an only child, with parents who did not happen to know or find congenial any other parents whatever with children of my own age, I don't remember ever playing with a child at home, in anyone else's home, in a 'swingie' (a playground with swings, roundabouts, seesaws, etc.) or anywhere.

A lot of my time was spent absorbing two sets, several volumes each, of an illustrated history of the world, and of an illustrated history of world literature. By the time I went to school I was beginning to read the texts of these encyclopaedias. Parts of literature and history are two subjects I've always felt I've always known but largely forgotten. Finding out about these things always felt as though I was simply refreshing my memory.

There would be words, however, that I had never known at all. When I had been at school for three months another closeted boy of my age, Walter Fyfe, who lived two houses down, came round (for the first and last time) for tea and cakes on a Sunday afternoon. We were each given some pieces to sight-read. I had a passage about a sailing ship which I found my way through not too badly. I pronounced the word 'boatswain' badly – 'boatswain' instead of 'bo'sun' – which Walter immediately pounced on, and I was in deep disgrace. I detested being subject to scorn and ridicule and 'you have let us down in front of Mrs Fyfe'. One of the feelings that the moment evoked vividly I found interesting later and still do. It was the feeling 'boatswain' and 'bo'sun' were expressions I had never come across before. Not like most other words I came across, spelled out, wrote down, looked up in the dictionary and wrote down the meaning of opposite the word in my own dictionary, which I compiled for years. Most words felt as though I had forgotten them, I once had known them. A word was like a familiar face I couldn't put a name to. But there were many words which on the other hand were much more remote. The vocabulary of plants, insects, architectural terms, as well as the vocabulary of the whole of recent science and technology.

All through my schooldays I assumed, and my parents, I think, assumed as well, that I would be around the top of my class. Indeed the other boys at the top of the class made the same assumption about themselves.

For three of the years I was at Cuthbertson's, I was in the same class as the headmaster's son. He was almost always first and I was second. There was no one else in the same league. None seemed to want to be, or felt they had to be, or tried to be, or in the least grudged us that position. And until I left the sixth form, there happened always to be two or three boys, of whom I was one, who were schoolboys in a very different way from the others, and there was also always another who, if not in every subject, would be the overall top.

My life was divided between school, home, music, Sunday School, and out playing.

I had virtually none of the bad experiences at school that mar so many people's lives. I savoured the company of most of my schoolmates and soon had several close friends. I was never brutalized, humiliated, degraded, savaged, raped, beaten up, bullied, and I never did anything like that to anyone else and never heard even a rumour of that happening to anyone else.

None of the masters were *serious* sadists. Several of them were feared because when they gave the strap they could really put themselves behind it and inflict a lot of pain with glee. But our school did not go as far as some. They could also give out long, long 'lines', and, what was the worst, were not always entirely predictable. Like at home, one knew the rules. If one broke them, one could expect lines or the strap – for talking in class, not paying attention, for running rather than walking inside the school building.

I had the record for two years, from twelve to thirteen, for being strapped in the 'Beak's' room, by the 'Beak' himself for 'running around' more than any other boy. Touch toes, knees straight, six of the best with the shredded end of a heavy, black leather strap across the bottom.

No, I don't think I was into a masochistic number. There were several packs of us who went pretty wild at 'intervals' or 'breaks' and hunted and chased each other through fascinating labyrinths of the old school building. I think I got caught six times in two years, several others were caught at least four times. It was a mark of distinction.

I suppose the penalty had to be sufficiently painful to be a deterrent. And it just about was. We had only a small playground. It was often raining, and anyway we spent 'intervals' as much in our classrooms as in the playground, so play went on inside or outside the school building. But inside it had to be subdued. Outside in the playground, there was never any issue. Inside was a limit. To break the limit meant six of the best. I dash around a corner 'not looking where I am going' and 'barge into' a teacher. 'Report to the Headmaster's room for six of the best right away.'

The last time the Beak stopped me he added, 'And next time I'll have to tell your father.' He said it rather routinely as though dictating a serious PS, but he caught a look of fear come into my eyes as he said it and to my surprise I glimpsed in his what I took to be a look as if to say, 'I'm sorry. I went too far. I didn't know,' and he added quickly, 'I hope that won't be necessary.' One way or another it wasn't.

The only way to keep out of trouble was to give up that sort of wildness completely, and I did, at the age of thirteen. With most of my friends. It was too painful. We settled for being well behaved and well out of trouble. There was no double bind entailed. If one behaved in a certain sort of way (and one knew what that certain sort of way was very well, and whether any particular behaviour was of that sort or not), then, if one got caught (and one was always liable to get caught, although comparatively seldom), one was punished. If one did not get caught, or did not behave in that sort of way one was not punished. The only way not to get punished was not to get caught. And the only way not to get caught every so often, every too often until once more is too often, is not to be doing anything one could be caught doing. From thirteen to seventeen that became my (and my friends') strategy. And it worked to everyone's satisfaction. I became an even better boy.

I am struck, looking back, at how sensitively the growth and development of our intellectual factors were canalized into those streams called subjects, 'Mathematics', 'Greek', 'Latin', 'Geography', 'History', 'Drawing', 'Gymnastics', 'English'. We had different teachers, usually for each subject. And how sensitive my mind was (and others' minds must be, as I know from my professional experience) to both the grossest pressures and slightest nuances of demands placed on it, and by whom. I shall never be sure whether I was never any good at geography because I disliked my geography teacher, or whether I disliked him because I disliked geography. I was never sure. Unlike history and English, the subject did not seem 'to come back' to me. I felt I had to learn it all for the first time like, later, anatomy.

As that seemed to be the state of mind of all but four or five of the others at the top of the class, about *all* subjects, there was no problem at all for us six to be at the top.

Mathematics is my main regret from my schooldays. I had one mathematics teacher till the end of the third year called 'the Bull', and 'Hutch' from fourth through to sixth. I was going along fine until 'the Bull' left, and suddenly I was plunged into mathematical idiocy. I could calculate arithmetically, but often made mistakes. And I could not understand what I was doing. I could not understand multiplication, division, even addition. I could not understand how the distance between two infinitely divisible points could be said to be the same as the distance between any two points. Worse still I could not understand what a

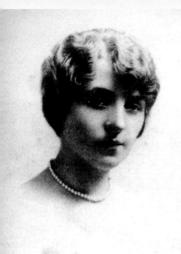

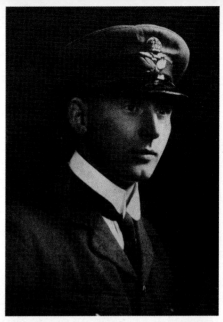

Above: Wedding portraits of my mother and father – Amelia Elizabeth (née Kirkwood) and David Park McNair Laing. My father is wearing the uniform of a lieutenant of the Royal Air Corps (the precursor of the RAF).

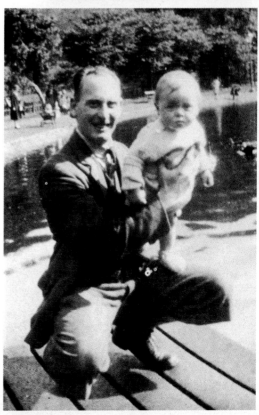

Right: My father and I at Queens Park Boating Pond, Glasgow, in 1927.

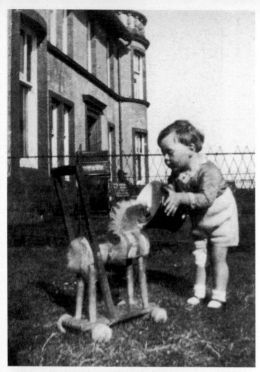

Left: I was very fond of this little wooden horse. Shortly after this photograph was taken at Troon, Ayrshire, my mother decided I was getting too fond of it and burned it.

Below left and below: My father often used to take me for walks in Glasgow's beautiful parks. These two photographs show me aged about four or five.

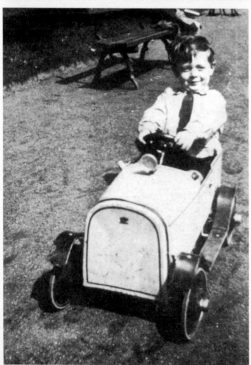

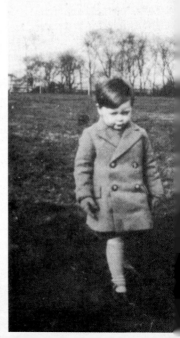

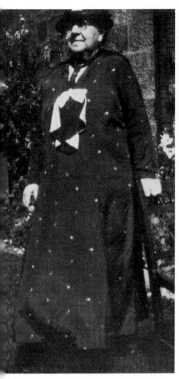

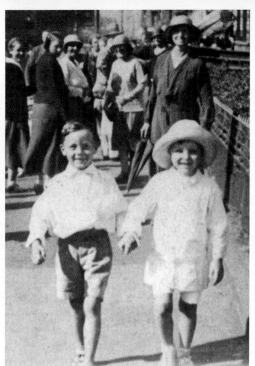

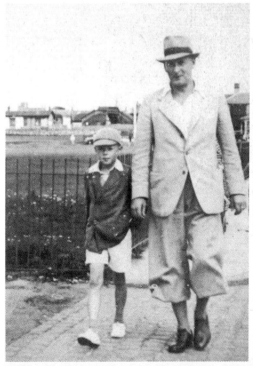

Above: Grannie, my mother's mother, photographed in 1934.

Top right: Me *(left)* with a cousin. Behind us is my aunt, my mother's elder sister.

Right: My father and I at Prestwick, Ayrshire, with the 'Royal and Ancient' Golf Club in the background. For years we used to play a round of golf in the morning, swim in the afternoon and have another nine holes in the evening. I have not played a complete round of golf since our last together over thirty years ago.

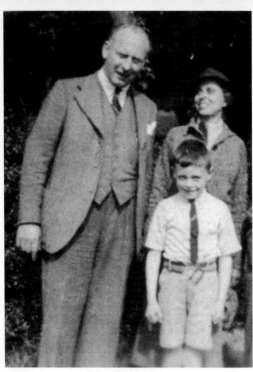

Left: My father, Gladys and I. For several years Gladys was my father's piano accompanist.

Below left: Portrait taken when I was about eleven.

Below: At the Bellahouston Engineering Exhibition, Glasgow, 1938.

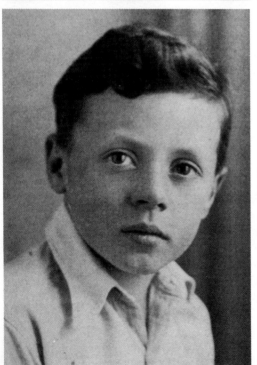

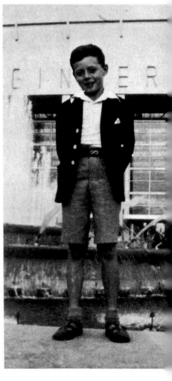

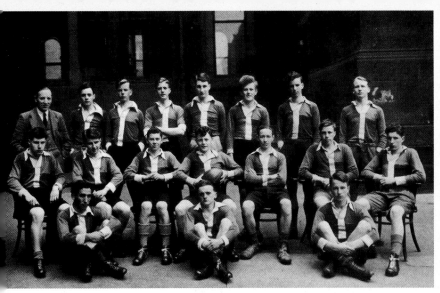

Hutcheson's Boys' Grammar School second rugby XV, 1943-44. (I am standing next to the teacher in the back row.) I was then in the fifth form. I never made the first XV, but I started playing rugby again when I joined the Army.

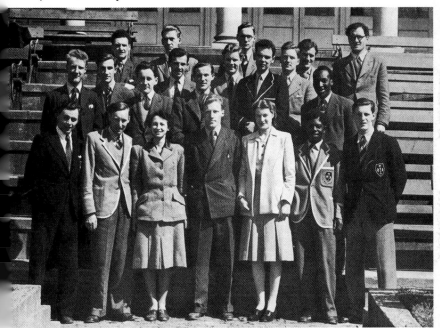

Glasgow University Athletics Team, 1945-46. (I am on the left of the front row.) As a first-year student I ran cross-country, but I then developed asthma and that brought my running career to an end after only one season.

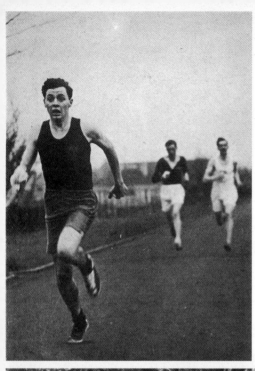

Left: Winning a cross-country run for Glasgow against Belfast University. My asthma began shortly after this and the first attack that knocked me out completely occurred, in fact, while I was running a race.

Below: Hitching in the Lake District with a friend during my student days.

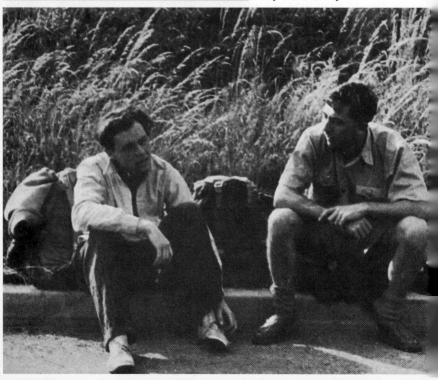

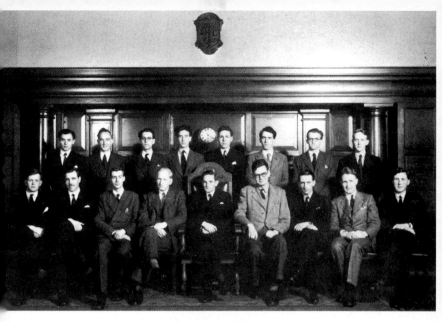

Glasgow University Medico-Chirurgical Society Committee,
1948-49. (I am on the left of the back row.)

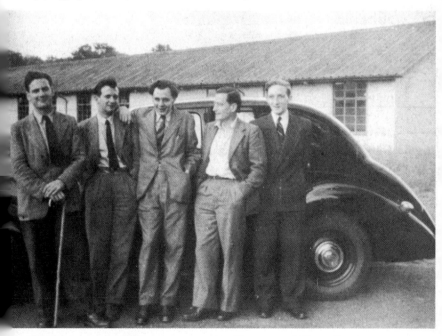

Myself (*centre*) and fellow interns at the Glasgow and West of
Scotland Neurosurgical Unit, Killearn, in 1951. The car belonged to
Joe Schorstein.

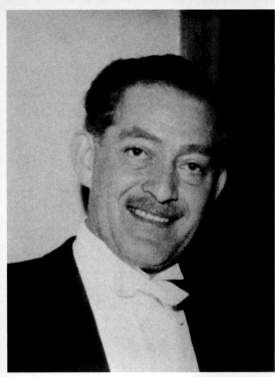

Left: Joe Schorstein, who became my medical mentor at the Neurosurgical Unit at Killearn.

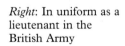

Right: In uniform as a lieutenant in the British Army

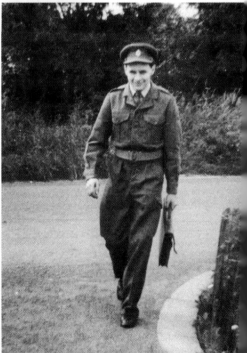

number *was*. What is a number? I kept on trying to imagine what a number was but there are unimaginable numbers. And so on. It was a terrible nightmare and I was so relieved when I sat my last paper in mathematics and never again had to put my mind through such real mental pain, perplexity, bewilderment.

It was not for twenty years, till I met one of the world's top mathematicians, David George Spencer-Brown, that I realized that the questions I was asking are precisely the sort of questions that are truly mathematical and that indeed mathematics at every step reveals more and more how mysterious a subject it is.

The ability truly not to understand what is taken for granted is the beginning of scientific or philosophical sagacity. It is a pity its manifestations are often greeted with ridicule, impatience, contempt, punishment. How stupid can you be in the fifth form not to know what a number is, much less not know how differences between them could be the same or different?

I could have got caught in such questions with every subject. But I regard myself as extremely fortunate I did not start having to ask what is grammar or what is a word or even a letter until I had no more exams to pass.

Until I passed my Diploma of Psychological Medicine in Glasgow in 1955, aged twenty-seven, which was the youngest age I could possibly have passed it, the main mental skill I had learned and become proficient in was how to pass exams. My only worry was that I might fail.

When I was fourteen my class had to write a home essay about ourselves. Mine began 'Time lies heavily on my hands.' My parents were very upset by this because they said it reflected on them. And anyway, they said, it doesn't. How could it? You are making it up. You always have plenty to do, school, homework, books, music, tennis, golf. You play rugby. How can you tell us that 'time lies heavily on your hands'? And it shows how ungrateful you are for all we have

done for you, and for how lucky you are. You do not realize
how privileged you are. So I changed the opening to 'I find
life full of interest' and went on to catalogue all the interesting things I was learning, like Greek irregular verbs and
Homer and Chopin, rugby, golf and tennis. They were
happy and I got a 'very good' and eight and a half out of ten.

That sort of deception, dissimulation, compliance some
people seem to find intolerable.

Also, one may have been deep-programmed, as I was,
against *living*, and here I was expected to lie, and of course
not let on at all that I was lying, or else – ? Or else it was
going to be very unpleasant. Such obstinacy in a fourteen-
year-old might call for a consultation with a psychiatrist
today, and he or she might be lucky enough to find a
sympathetic psychiatrist or psychologist in whom he or she
could confide without having to worry that it would be held
against one, in some way, if one told the truth quite
candidly about how one felt about life.

I am very glad now I bent with the wind then and later. I
think asthma was one of the prices I had to pay for my sense
of suffocation and my policy of doing my best to keep out of
trouble, just for the sake of a quiet life.

I just had to live with the most unpleasant queasy sense of
corruption. It is terrible to feel you have to pretend you love
someone when you do not.

I was out for a stroll with my father about thirty years ago.
My oldest daughter was just beginning to toddle. She
toddled a few steps ahead of us on her own and fell down.
I ran forward and picked her up. My father turned to me
and said, 'You know, your mother would have given you a
good spanking for that.'

I do not remember those days myself, but my father's
remark fits with my feeling that if I fall down, in any way,
I've done something wrong, it's my fault, and I will, or will
deserve, to be punished for it. It's still my fault if I catch the
'flu; or it is to teach me something: maybe that it's not my
fault.

THE FIRE AND THE STREET

Those were the days of coal fires, draughty windows and doors. Every evening every winter, after piano practice, work and some reading for fun, I would curl up in front of the fire and gaze into it for half an hour or so before going to bed.

As I looked at the fire I became absorbed in it and faded away into it. I was wide awake. It was not the same as going to sleep. I took it as much for granted as going to sleep. I could equally say I took sleep as much for granted as gazing-into-the-fire. Years later I was very surprised to find that this process, this fading away awake through empty-minded, bare attention is a widely cultivated form of meditation.

I used to sit near my mother for long hours, gazing out of the window at the street. I spent as much time looking out of the window as my children spend watching TV.

The window was as a one-way screen.

Liking fading into the fire, it was only years later that I discovered that there was a special branch of social science devoted to what I had been looking at, and that this empty-minded, bare, absorbed attention to what was happening was called 'vipassana meditation'. It was the best possible preparation I could have had for what later became apparent was one of my central interests – human interaction.

The hours and years some children spent birdwatching, I spent watching people.

And how the mood and character of the street changed, as it grew dusk, as the men came home from work and the streets emptied and the gaslighter went round lighting up each lamp in turn, one by one; the shops began to close and people pulled their curtains to, their blinds down and eventually sat round the fire watching those 'blue-bleak embers, ah my dear, Fall, gall themselves, and gash gold-vermilion.'* And then to bed.

* From Gerard Manley Hopkins, 'The Windhover'.

How do I know what I can do? Can I make someone walking by look up at me? Can I make someone walk faster or slower? Can I make the gaslights dimmer or brighter? Can I make the flames in the fire leap? higher? or lower? Can I . . . ?

The people in the street were not toys like my tin soldier. I had not found out how to turn people into puppets, but maybe . . . ? Once someone turned round and looked right at me looking at him, a tiny face, resting on a window sill, out of a dark room, one up. More than once I seemed to dance with the flames.

My life-saving consolations were moonlight and gaslight, the angel on the dome of the library, music, the coal fire, fun, indeed all things – sky, sun, stars, clouds, rain, sleep, snow, flowers, trees, birds, flies, prayer, a few people, even asphalt, fog. . . . What the hell was the matter with us? Why did we not join the rest of creation, and all have a great time on this glorious jewel of a planet together? No. Nothing remotely like it. Why not? In God's name why not?

My mother did not sing me lullabies but she taught me to say prayers.

Almost fifty years later, after my father was dead, I asked her whether she believed in any of that sort of thing – 'It's all a lot of nonsense, Ronald.'

MUSIC

There was always music. My mother played the piano and my father sang, and people came round to the house to make music.

I can't remember in my whole childhood being in the presence of any roomful of adults who had met simply to sit around and talk except at Old Pa's at New Year when the company was confined to the family: Old Pa, Ethel, Jack, my father, my mother, Wee Johnny. One of the chief pleasures in life later has been just to sit around with friends, smoking, drinking, talking about this or that, or about life, or not, or a tight argument, or a close-knit conversation, or the very *in* talking of professionals imbued with their own subject.

There was none of that at home or elsewhere as a child, but I didn't miss it – I amply made up for it later – and instead there was music: more than a fair exchange. If I had to choose either talking or singing, it would have to be singing. Talking seemed simply deteriorated singing, singing without much melody, timbre, rhythm or pitch. Just music gone flat, rotten, dead. Yes, singing and music were *alive*.

My father had always sung in the choir. When he came out of the Royal Air Corps as a lieutenant at the end of World War I, his ambition was to become principal baritone at Covent Garden. He didn't make it to there, but became a respected part-time professional, for the club, the social, the radio broadcast. He had not the voice for the theatre. And he was the principal baritone at the Glasgow University Chapel Choir. The organist and choirmaster was A. M. Henderson, a distinguished musician, who had studied with Widor, and wrote two books of memoirs about his friendships with Albert Schweitzer, Rachmaninov, Scriabin, and others in the musical firmament. So I heard at home before I was born my father practising the baritone parts of the full accomplished choir repertoire and the usual repertoire of a professional baritone with a penchant for Italian opera and Victorian ballads. Nothing more modern than Roger Quilter, however.

It wasn't the musical Big Time, but it was on the fringe of it, and the musicians I heard were good enough sometimes to reverberate that physical resonance to beauty that produces a shiver, or a quiver, makes some people fibrillate, some people get an ache in their throat, their eyes moisten, they cry or sob or whimper. I know several exquisitely musical people who can't go to a concert or listen to live music in any company other than the most relaxed where it is all right to show some emotion.

In some musical company I have been in, in Morocco, in India, it is a mark of distinction to be moved to tears at the appropriate moments. But it won't do at a concert in the West.

Anyway, when my father got on to wringing the heart out of a song, say 'None but the Lonely Heart' or even 'Roses of Picardy', the sound of his own voice would moisten his eyes, his nasal passages (so he might have to clear his nose between songs and produce a very fast flickering fibrillation of his cheeks) just when he entered that zone where one needs dry eyes as a performer to bring tears to the eyes of the listener.

I used to argue with my father about this. And I still think I am right. It would go something like this: 'Dad. It's a pity you lost the last bit of that Tchaikovsky. *We're* supposed to cry; *you* are supposed to be dry-eyed.'

'Yes. I know. I can't stop it. You've got to *feel* the song.'

In the first two years of my piano and music lessons, I had to do one hour of homework a day. I first had to learn to read off the names of notes until they came automatically (this took, I think, two or three weeks), then I had to learn them on the piano until that was almost automatic, then I was started off on my first pieces and scales.

I was not allowed to touch the piano keys unless I was playing something or practising scales or finger exercises. Every finger had to rest properly on each key and be depressed and lifted properly. Every single note I struck had to be struck with the correct finger. All notes of both hands were numbered one to five on each hand. I never ever played or practised without my father sitting beside me. He never let me go on if I ever played a wrong note or a note wrongly or with the wrong finger. When I came back from my music lesson I had to tell him exactly where my teacher, Julia, had corrected me in any way or told me anything new, and he wrote it all down in a diary he kept of my music lessons. Julia had very little to correct and I made such rapid progress that she let me 'do the fingering' myself.

In fact, my father did all the fingering and wrote it all out as Julia had done in pencil, a number for each note.

I was now on the foothills of the standard classical repertoire. Julia was very pre-emptory and twice when she stopped me abruptly and started me up again, my fingers started to quiver and my hands went into a horizontal tremor across the keys. She now would ask for 'more expression' but I could only play *pp*, *p*, *mf*, *f* or *ff*, *dim.* and *rall.* and so on as written, and 'That's your father's writing. Write out the fingering yourself.' I told her that father 'did the fingering'. She asked him to come to my next music lesson and after thanking him for taking such a great interest in Ronald's music lessons told him that she now wanted him to stop doing my fingering and to let me practise without him sitting over me, and I heard her say, 'Now, Mr Laing, I want to hear Ronald play the piano and not you.'

I had no idea what a relief it would be to hear her say what she did until she said it. It had not really occurred to me until I heard her explain it to my father, and I am sure it had not occurred to him either, to look at it that way. My father honoured her wishes with good grace, and I never found him intrusive.

I kept a diary going, writing in it 'religiously' until after one lesson I couldn't be bothered and didn't. My father saw that I hadn't written up the lesson and told me to do so. I said, 'Why should I?' and he landed me a swinging, full slap across my left cheek. 'Don't ever dare to use that tone of voice to me.'

We left it at that. I wrote up a few notes of the years thereafter, but basically that was the end of the diary.

When I was ten, I was thought to have perfect pitch. I was given several ear tests which seemed to confirm this view until I had one at which I failed miserably. It was decided that, in some undetected way, I must have been cheating. I was tested again and yet again and failed hopelessly each time. I was in awful disgrace.

I could never make up my own mind whether I had been

cheating or not. If I had been cheating, I did not know I
had. It had not occurred to me I might have perfect pitch,
until it was concluded I hadn't. My innocent confidence
was shattered.

They told me I had not got perfect pitch. They told me I
was a cheat. I had deceived them. I was agonized. I had to
believe them yet I could not believe them without completely abdicating my whole being. They thought I might
have perfect pitch. It had never occurred to me. I had never
thought about it. I had no convictions or pretensions.
When they struck a note I said the first note that occurred
to me and it was right. Of course Rachmaninov's Prelude in
C sharp Minor could not have been conceived in G Minor.
With no doubts and no convictions, my naïve guesses were
infallibly right. Then I lost my innocence. I began to think I
might and doubt that I did, and it was gone, or inaccessible
to me.

If I had been cheating, I wish I could have refound the
trick. Or perhaps I had lost either this gift or the trick, or
both. The magic had evaporated, and I was pierced by the
poisoned arrow of self-doubt.

The venom from this poisoned arrow of self-doubt made
me feel physically ill, leaked outside music, but was largely
contained in it. It wiped out my naïve trust in myself. Thus
I have drawn on my musical schizophrenia – this episode
induced in me a lot of my subsequent psychiatric studies. I
was once more hypnotized. I had perfect pitch. I was
ordered to believe that I had not. I was not a cheat. I
was ordered to believe I was. I could not believe them and I
could not disbelieve them. What does a mind do in such an
instance? Musically my internal tonal scheme was completely shattered. I was in doubt as to the difference
between a fifth and an octave. Ear tests were a nightmare.

I could not believe them and I would not believe them. I
both believed them and did not believe them. I was in a
quadralemma. Though I did not believe the belief, the belief
had a grip on my musical mental operations, at a level more

deep than my own disbelief in the belief could reach. That is being hypnotized.

My belief in the lack of perfect pitch required me to destroy the evidence of perfect pitch. So that if I had perfect pitch, it was no longer evident. Now, therefore, my belief in myself could not be based on the evidence of my senses. It could only be based on a belief that my sensibility was not evident. An unnerving position to have to cling to.

How could I ever know? How could I ever tell?

The whole rigmarole effectively destroyed any access to the perfect pitch I had. It is still tucked way back.

This experience and others have left me with the abiding feeling that there is something cracked about my musical mind.

A LONG-TERM PLAN

Sometime before I was born my mother had 'shut the piano lid' and vowed never to play for my father again. He had to find accompanists. After several years he found Gladys. Gladys had a wry neck (*torticollis*) and a club foot. She was a very devout High Anglican lady. She would often come round to the house and accompany David on Amelia's black baby grand Challen piano while Amelia sat and appreciated her playing, apparently ungrudgingly, and made tea.

During World War II Gladys regularly worked till ten at night in Paterson's Music Studios in Buchanan Street. It was the time of the black-out. My father would regularly go from Crosshill to Buchanan Street at twenty to nine by bus to collect Gladys, accompany her to her bus, travel with her to Burnside, walk her from the bus terminus to her bungalow and return home just after eleven.

Amelia did not seem to mind. It was very dark outside. She wouldn't like to be outside in the dark at that time of night through the winter at her age and, with a wry neck and club foot, she was just very lucky to have David who was such a gentleman when he put his mind to it.

Then something happened. Gladys said something to Amelia which Amelia would never repeat to anyone. Her eyes were opened.

Of course she could not say anything to David. David was really simple-minded, he could not see through someone like Gladys. If she said anything against Gladys he would only think she was jealous of her.

He would have to see for himself what Gladys was like. How? It took three years of biding her time before the solution presented itself.

We should all go for a week's holiday together. Yes. We've never done that before. An excellent idea. Two adjacent rooms in a boarding house on the front in Prestwick. Amelia and Gladys would have separate beds in one room, David and Ronald sleep in the other.

Fine. The first night there we went to our rooms. Amelia and Gladys put on their nightdresses and David and Ronald put on their pyjama suits. Ronald put on a nightgown as well. David never wore a nightgown.

And then, before turning in for the night, David and Ronald came through to say goodnight to Amelia and Gladys.

Gladys fell back on her bed in a faint. It was not serious. She soon recovered. She did not know what had come over her. We all hoped it would be all right, Gladys was sure it was, we said goodnight and went to bed.

Next day Gladys was not entirely better and she felt she had better go home – which she did.

David could not understand why Gladys had fainted.

'Whatever came over Gladys?' he asked Amelia the next day. Amelia reserved for this question one of her most special expressions, which might crudely be translated to signify something like this: 'How can you be so incredibly stupid as to ask such a question? If you don't know by now no one can tell you. With all your brains and your intelligence you know nothing. You would be much better not to pursue the matter. Go on living in your own fool's paradise. I am not saying anything.'

David was completely hooked. It took a lot of persistence to get it out of Amelia.

'I've told you so often.'

'What?'

'About your *pyjamas*.'

'What's wrong with my pyjamas?'

'You don't realize that Gladys is a *lady*.'

My father insisted that Gladys would not be shocked by anything like that – but the point had been made. He could not dismiss it.

He saw less of Gladys. He no longer enjoyed singing with her. He stopped seeing her.

'Your mother is a most astute woman. She is a most astute judge of character. I must say she opened my eyes to Gladys. I never realized that Gladys was like that.'

The whole story could be entirely my imagination. Not a word was spoken about any of it, in my presence, except what I have put down. I shall never know. Nevertheless, supposing I was right. Supposing I was right, what went on in that bedroom in a flash, for a few seconds, derived its meaning from a tissue of entirely silent manipulation, going on for years. Only one person could know if this were true and she would never tell. She might as well say she had been spinning her web for years to catch Gladys, as she might deny it. 'Ronald, we never talk about that sort of thing.' Hence I became fascinated by all those sorts of things we don't talk about.

THE BATH

Naturally I was expected to keep myself clean. It was usual to have a hot bath every night and, in the winter, a cold bath in the morning.

In my fifteenth year the bath became a dreadful experience. My mother had always rubbed my back. The area she rubbed and the length of time taken to do so had dwindled until it was little more than a spot in the middle between my shoulders, and only for a few seconds. Nevertheless she had to come into the bathroom to do this.

I was concerned that when she did so she might catch a glimpse of my recently sprouting pubic hair, so I made myself sufficiently dirty in some not-so-obvious way (otherwise I would have had to wash it beforehand) so that the bathwater would be opaque.

The details of the procedure were the outcome of negotiation between my mother and me. She refused to allow me to lock the bathroom door. I had the right to call her in when I was ready. She was on her honour not to come in before she was called, just to perform the necessary, and to leave.

The ostensible reason for all this was that I was not able to clean all of my back properly myself, and if this one area were left improperly cleaned, a spot might appear there and be the beginning of another new type of rash.

I found this arrangement more and more humiliating. Finally I locked the door. My mother stood outside beating on the frosted glass. She quickly escalated from yelling (Open this door at once. Come on now. This is your mother. Open this door.) to even higher pitched yells and screams through which she threatened to break the door down.

At this point, my father dragged her away from the door. The yelling and screaming were unabated and her intention persisted. He remonstrated with her to no effect. Then he yelled at her yell for yell, 'If you don't stop it, I'll go out on the stairhead and shout my bloody head off!' The neighbours! That did it. She quietened down. I was already out of the bathroom.

I was deeply grateful to my father that when it came to the crunch he took my side. It would have been awful if he too had ordered me to open the door.

THE ACCIDENT

Cycling along a street in the Gorbals, Glasgow. Children are playing as usual in the middle of the road. A boy of

maybe five or six dashes across the path of my bike. I knock
him down and my bike and I fall apart on to the road. I pick
myself up. It wasn't my fault. Several women are running to
the boy and are beginning to pick him up. The women are
picking the boy up. He is starting to howl. Thank God – he
can't be severely injured. I am not hurt, I think. I cry out to
the women.

'It's not my fault. He ran in front of me. I couldn't do
anything.'

One of them turns to me. 'It's all right. I saw it. It's not
your fault.'

I stay a little, so I won't be thought to be dawdling off too
callously, and then cycle away.

I think this happened the winter after I was converted.

The incident arrested my attention and has stayed vividly
in my mind's eye. It showed me as clearly as possible that in
an emergency, when I was simply reacting, I had no
immediate concern for the boy whatever.

If he was hurt it would be trouble for me, even if it wasn't
my fault. The first things that occurred to me were:

1. I'm in the clear. It isn't my fault.
2. Is he seriously hurt? He can't be dead. No. I hope
   he isn't seriously hurt because that will be a real
   nuisance to me even if no one blames me.
3. Is the bike all right?
4. I am *exonerated* – what a relief – no one was
   blaming me.
5. How soon can I get out of it?
6. Only when driving away, breathing freely, did a
   feeling occur to me of relief on the boy's behalf.
   'I'm glad he's OK.'

That being 'glad' *he* was OK was a totally different feeling
from being 'glad' *I* was OK because *he* seemed OK, and
anyway it wasn't my fault.

I'm still 'glad' all round.

The incident brought home to me that there was within me no genuine altruism, but that my dominant feelings were entirely self-serving and full of fear – if not abject cowardice.

1. I was afraid of being blamed. In that neighbourhood I might well have been set upon and beaten up, but even apart from that

2. I was afraid of being subject to my own sense of blame. If I had felt it was my fault I would still have tried to get away with it and I think I would rather have got away with it, although guilty, than have been blamed by them, though I knew I was innocent.

This incident epitomizes for me the state of my original heart. 'As pure as the driven slush.'

It seemed far deeper than anything 'I' could do about it. 'I' was in fact the very heart of that ego-centred system. What was it that made me feel that I was rotten? No more rotten than others. Just *as* rotten as the rest of the people I knew.

Only a miracle could change this state of affairs. Only the Grace of the Lord Jesus Christ. All I could do, and that only by his Grace, was to pray for Mercy – and whatever, in whatever event, Thy will be done. As it was being done anyway. No evil is done in the city unless I do it, saith the Lord.

WHAT TO BELIEVE?

The first two prizes I won were at Sunday School: a prize for a year's perfect attendance and perfect conduct, never absent, never late, never 'checked' for anything, and a prize for reciting with no hesitations or mistakes the books of the Bible from *Genesis* through to *Revelation* the fastest in my class. (*Deep breath*) Genesis Exodus Leviticus Numbers Deuteronomy Joshua Judges Ruth First Samuel Second

Samuel First Kings Second Kings First Chronicles Second
Chronicles Ezra Nehemiah Esther Job Psalms Proverbs
Ecclesiastes Song of Solomon Isaiah Jeremiah Lamenta-
tions Ezekiel Daniel Hosea Joel Amos Obadiah Jonah
Micah Nahum Habakkuk (*breath*) Zephaniah Haggai Ze-
chariah Malachi (*the hardest line, easy when you get it, deep
breath, then home and dry*) Matthew Mark Luke John Acts
Romans First Corinthians Second Corinthians Galatians
Ephesians Philippians Colossians First Thessalonians Sec-
ond Thessalonians First Timothy Second Timothy Titus
Philemon Hebrews James First Peter Second Peter First
John Second John Third John Jude Revelation (*forty seconds*).

I was four. I was sent to Sunday School a year earlier than
to primary school. At Sunday School we sang hymns, read
the Bible, learned by heart passages from it and the Short
Catechism of the Westminster Divines, said prayers.

> *Question*: What is the chief end of Man?
> *Answer*: Man's chief end is to glorify God, and to
> enjoy Him for ever.

There are one hundred and seven questions and answers to
be memorized and believed in with one's eternal salvation
or damnation at stake. Here are samples:

> *Q4*: What is God?
> *A*: God is Spirit, infinite, eternal, and unchangeable,
> in His being, wisdom, power, holiness, justice,
> goodness, and truth.

But:

> *Q2*: What rule hath God given to direct us how we may
> glorify and enjoy Him?
> *A*: The Word of God, which is contained in the
> scriptures of the Old and New Testaments, is the
> only rule to direct us how we may glorify and enjoy
> Him.

Q15: What was the sin whereby our first parents fell from the estate wherein they were created?

A: The sin whereby our first parents fell from the estate wherein they were created was their eating forbidden fruit.

Q16: Did all mankind fall in Adam's first transgression?

A: The covenant being made with Adam, not only for himself, but for his posterity, all mankind, descending from him, by ordinary generation, sinned in him, and fell with him, in his first transgression.

Q17: Into what estate did the fall bring mankind?

A: The fall brought mankind into an estate of sin and misery.

Q18: Wherein consists the sinfulness of that estate whereinto Man fell?

A: The sinfulness of that estate whereinto Man fell consists in the guilt of Adam's first sin, the want of original righteousness, and the corruption of his whole nature, which is commonly called Original Sin; together with all actual transgressions which proceed from it.

Q19: What is the misery of that estate whereinto Man fell?

A: All mankind by their fall lost communion with God, are under his wrath and curse, and so made liable to all miseries in this life, to death itself, and to the pains of Hell forever.

That is us, that is our lot, but:

Q20: Did God leave all mankind to perish in the estate of sin and misery?

A: God having, out of His mere good pleasure, from

all eternity, elected some to everlasting life, did
enter into a covenant of grace, to deliver them out
of the estate of sin and misery, and to bring them
into an estate of salvation by a Redeemer.

Every word in the English Bible was true. It all came from
God. It was God's Holy Book. It was His Word. To
disobey it was to disobey God, to be in grievous sin.

I said my prayers every night, sitting up in bed before
going to sleep, eyes shut, head bowed, hands together. I
can't remember ever not saying my prayers until I was
seventeen.

As I lay me down to sleep,
I pray the Lord my soul to keep.
If I should die before I wake,
I pray the Lord my soul to take.
God bless Mummy and Daddy and wee Ronnie and make
wee Ronnie a good boy for Jesus' sake Amen.

The clause 'If I should die before I wake, I pray the Lord
my soul to take' was alarming. Supposing I died while I was
away in the depth of sleep, would God be looking, would
He notice, would I be lost forever? But if I did not forget to
remind Him, He would not forget to remember. So everything was all right.

When my father was fourteen an angel had appeared to
him while he was lying awake in bed one night and kissed
him on the forehead. I never asked him and he never told
me what it looked like. He believed that its kiss had blessed
his whole life. I never saw an angel.

We were Presbyterians. The only persons I knew who were
not were Gladys, my father's accompanist, an Episcopa-
lian, and Julia Ommer, my music teacher, who was a
Roman Catholic.

We knew no Jews. They have different germs from us.
Auntie Maisie had gone into a Jewish house when she was

twelve and got a Jewish germ. That was why she was deaf in her left ear.

The Jews had been God's chosen people. Chosen to be held as an example to the world. They had crucified Christ. What was happening to them was what they had brought upon themselves. They were different from us. And they knew it. They smelt differently. I should not sit beside a Jewish boy at school. If the teacher insisted, and he wouldn't, I should tell him. He would understand. Jews should not be allowed to stink out the local fish shop. Fresh herrings from Aberdeen had a Jewish smell in a few hours on a Friday morning. They ought to keep to themselves. They should have their own shops.

'About the only thing to be said for Hitler,' I heard a woman say in the street, as Glasgow was being bombed, 'is that he is finishing them off,' and, later, the only trouble with the war ending when it did was that 'he didn't have a chance to finish the job.'

Every morning at general assembly in my boys' grammar school, the Rector sang the following hymn:

> God be in my head and in my understanding
> God be in my eyes and in my looking
> God be in my mouth and in my speaking
> God be in my heart and in my thinking
> God be at my end and at my departing.

One of the prefects read out one or two dozen verses from the Bible, and the whole school, masters and boys, recited the Lord's Prayer together.

I often repeated these prayers to myself. I had seriously sinned by breaking my promise and lying over the sweeties. God alone could save me and I prayed He would do so, and behaved myself. That was all I could do. But I never felt I was saved.

We had a religious class at school, one hour a week. When I was fourteen this class began to be taken by

'Fergie', a teacher who called himself an agnostic. Instead of giving us religious instruction as at Sunday School, he got us to discuss what we believed and what we did not believe. He was a 'free thinker'. The Bible was not necessarily true. He did not believe there was a God, though he could not prove there was not, so he preferred to call himself an agnostic rather than an atheist. He did not believe he was going to be damned because he did not believe in the Lord Jesus Christ. There were many wise men and people who did not believe in God. Socrates and Gandhi were not Christians. The Buddha was an atheist. There was no life after death.

This was the first time I ever heard such sacrilegious and blasphemous views. Some parents objected to Fergie's classes but the Rector, the 'Beak', who professed to be a Christian himself, upheld the view that a religious class could be an open enquiry into what was right belief and conduct.

It transpired that my father's father was a Spencerian, an evolutionist, a materialist, an ethical humanist, an avowed agnostic, and possibly an atheist.

My father turned out to be a very ambiguous believer. We would argue for hours a day for three or four years over God.

If God is good why does He allow all the awful things that go on? This is an unfathomable mystery. Many things are not revealed. We see through a glass very darkly.

God helps them who help themselves. I won a bet of half-a-crown with my father that this was not in the Bible. I read the Bible from cover to cover without coming across it.

Does God exist? Yes, said my father. And what is God? He is the idealized conception of Man's own image. Then you are an atheist. Not at all.

They had told me they were Santa Claus. Now my father was virtually telling me that he was God. I did not want to believe him.

The Scripture Union, Crusaders and Covenanters were

all strong in our school. I was a member of all three, but I did not feel I was 'converted' till I was fifteen, at a school camp.

We listened every night to the Gospel story recounted in twelve dramatic instalments by a Church of Scotland Minister called the 'Boss' for the express purpose of converting boys to Christ. On the twelfth night, I gave in.

I told the 'Boss' I had chosen the Lord Jesus Christ. You have not chosen Christ. Christ, he prayed, had chosen me. Christ alone knew.

As quickly as I had felt 'converted', I felt unconverted. I longed to feel converted but I couldn't. I went to Scripture Union Meetings and played the organ at Sunday School, prayed, kept my innocence, but did not know any more what I believed or what to believe. At that same time I believed that what I or anyone 'believed' was somehow vitally important, more important than what one thought, or felt. What one believed our life and death to be was, in all senses, truly a matter of life and death.

I read the sceptics, Epictetus, Montaigne, Voltaire, Marx, Nietzsche; I became a sort of nihilist, atheistic, dialectical, historical, materialist, Freudian, communist anarchist.

The trouble with Jesus, I told the 'Boss' a year later in my farewell conversation with him, was they got Him too young. He didn't have time to mature like the Buddha. He said I was a fool. He said he would pray for me and suggested I read Karl Barth.

I started off believing, I think, everything I was told. I believed because I had been told it. But I did not want to go through life believing what I had been told because I had been told it.

Did masturbation produce acne, sap one's moral fibre and lead to softening of the brain? I did not believe it did, but it still took courage to find out for myself. Was sexual intercourse sinful outside marriage? This question cannot be put to the test in the same way. The fact that I could fornicate without feeling guilty about it might only go to show how depraved I had become.

I fell away rapidly. I swore once or twice. I listened to a dirty joke. I told a dirty joke. I could see nothing against masturbation or sexual intercourse or dance music. I went to a music shop and exposed myself, trembling, to jazz for the first time, *ever*, aged sixteen. I looked at nudes in books in bookshops. I smoked a few cigarettes. Two years later I got drunk. I sang blasphemous words to hymn tunes. I knew prayers were being said for me.

When I was eighteen, as I learned from my mother when I was twenty-one, her mother, Grannie, had come round to our house – 'the first time she had set foot in the door for sixteen years' – to tell my mother she had had a dream that 'Ronald has gone evil'.

Grannie and Mummy had not shared the awful truth with anyone that I had 'gone evil'. When my mother revealed this fact to me I assumed she still believed it.

THREE

University

At the end of my schooldays I had to take stock, of where I was at, and where I was going. My parents left the choice of what to do up to me.

In some ways my most facile talent seemed to be music. I had been offered a scholarship at the Royal Academy of Music in London when I was twelve, but that was 'impossible because of the war'. When I was sixteen, playing rugby one frosty Saturday morning, my left wrist was crushed into the frost and was fractured in eight places. That finished off my left hand for almost a year, but nevertheless before I left school I had become an Associate of the Royal College of Music (ARCM) and a Licentiate of the Royal Academy of Music (LRAM). A musical career was still not out of the question. But I ruled it out as a primary career. I kept on piano lessons, now with A. M. Henderson, organist at the Glasgow University Chapel. I taught the piano at the Ommer Academy of Music. There are two or three music teachers in Glasgow who were once my pupils. I accompanied the occasional singing teacher at small-time concerts, was in demand at parties and played in small ensembles, at weddings, receptions, composed a few tunes. I kept it up but I had to reconcile myself to it becoming more of a consolation than my central activity in life.

When I left school my classics teacher told me that I had a comfortable MA-level of competence in Greek and Latin. I did not want to let them slip away, but I had not enough love for these languages and their literature as far as I had tasted them to want to devote myself to them for the rest of my life: nor to languages as such, nor to pure scholarship or teaching or preaching.

I was very imbued with books. Right outside my bedroom window was the dome of a public library on the top of which was an angel, poised on one foot, as though to take off to the moon and the stars.

I had started eating my way through the library from A to Z after I broke my left wrist and my arm was in plaster for months, so that not only could I not play the piano with it but I could not run, play rugby, golf, cycle. I read. This way I first came across Freud, Kierkegaard, Marx and Nietzsche. Somewhere among what they were going on about lay my obsessions. I was so grateful for books, for libraries, for the writers of such books, for the endowers and organizers of public libraries. I wanted to be a writer. Or rather, I was convinced I *was* a writer, like them, and that it was my duty, my necessity, to become the writer I was. I gave myself the age of thirty as an absolute deadline for the publication of my first book.

But I knew I was going to have to be very fortunate and to keep on working very hard, and even to accelerate, if I was going to have anything to say. I was sure that I could write, but I was not sure when I would have anything I felt justified to write about.

I knew what I wanted to write about. I wanted to ferret out some sort of truth about what was going on in the human world. What the truth was to be I would not know till it dawned on me. Why was the human race so unhappy? Why did we all have to die? The pity of it. Was it really going to be as it seemed it could not help but be – poisons, plagues, the Bomb, irradiation, sickness, death or a fate worse than death? What was the trouble? What was the matter? What the hell was going on?

Human sin, said the Christians; capitalism, said the Marxists. It could not be summed up in a word or a few words. In any event, I realized that all I knew about the human scene was a family, a few streets, a school, a Sunday

School, a church, a few musicians, rigorously censored music, a few books, the radio, the inside of a railway compartment once a year and the sea from the sand and a few roads and places in Scotland. Beyond such few scraps, I was totally ignorant.

I could read books and write them anyway. I did not need, I felt, to learn anything at university as to what and how to read or what or how to write. No one was ever going to make me sit another examination on that.

What is suffering? Why are we suffering in the way we are? Why did people seem to be so cruel? Maybe I could answer such questions, partially.

Medicine fell into place. If I went into medicine I would learn to be scientific. I would be addressing myself to real physical, material reality – birth, death, disease, pain – and to real social realities – poverty and pestilence – and within the warps in the brain I might find the cause of the warps in the mind.

My undergraduate medical training at Glasgow University consisted of two pre-clinical and three clinical years. One year of physics, chemistry, botany and biology. One year of anatomy and physiology. Then the clinical years of general medicine, surgery and the other major divisions of ortho-dox Western medicine.

I became scaldingly aware of my own complete ignor-ance of every subject I was being taught. How was I ever going to catch up? How was I ever going to get to the growing point, the cutting edge? At the rate they, my teachers, seemed to be going, they seemed to be widening the gap between me, or any starting student, and them, every day. They had been keeping up their pace for years. How many years would it take me, going all out, to get up alongside them and go beyond them? It all, I felt, would be an utter waste of time if I could not or did not 'make it' to the growing edge, the starting line.

I had flashes of how terrible it would be at the age of

thirty or forty, if I lived that long, to look back at myself at the age of twenty and rebuke that young man I was for his self-indulgence, sloth, frivolity, dalliance, debauchery, depravity, and miscalculation, stupidity, lack of sagacity, as well.

I had to discharge a duty to myself of twenty or more years older. I had to put in the groundwork now to give myself a chance later, even the faintest chance, of being in a position to make any possible 'contribution' of any moment or substance in any field.

Our anatomy professor, Professor Hamilton, and his assistant Dr Harrison, were the first to stir me with the passion for research.

Harrison impressed on me that it was impossible to get anywhere in research with over six hours' sleep a night, absolute maximum. He had cut down to between two and three hours by reducing the time he slept by five minutes a night with the aid of an alarm clock. I once fell asleep in the front row of an anatomy lecture given by Professor Hamilton. He prodded me awake with his long lecture pointer, but later commended me that I was 'down to five'.

I once ventured to ask Professor Hamilton what was his ambition as an embryologist. He began to froth at the mouth. I have not seen exactly the same phenomenon before or since. He was frothing with urgency and fervour. He could not be an Einstein. He could not even be a Newton. Embryology was at a stage of its own embryological development. Compared to physics it was pre-Newtonian. All he could do was keep on filling in the gaps in the total description of embryological development. There were still many, many gaps in our knowledge of the detailed chronology of the cellular changes of form and function in human embryological development. He could offer some more pieces to the vast jigsaw of data coming in from the whole of comparative embryology, genetics, and so on. He wished me luck with my desire to study the mind scientifically. But he said he thought I would be prudent to take on something simpler, like embryology. If I had had enough mathematical talent to study embryology from the vantage point of theoretical physics, I think I would have had a go at being an embryologist. But, without mathematics, I felt I would be more prudent to address myself to a field I could look at and study scientifically, and to which I could make a valid contribution, without mathematics.

Hamilton had no interest in the motives that drive one into scientific research. The crux of science was the scientific method, not why, or what, but how. He respected the painstaking work of a German anatomist, a fundamentalist Christian, on the comparative microstructure of the retina between primates and humans, who wanted to discredit Darwinian and post-Darwinian evolution by showing that *microscopically* the retinas of primates and humans were built on a different plan.

It was very encouraging to me that Hamilton did not discourage me from becoming interested in hypnotism even though it was a far cry from embryology. As long as I kept to the scientific straight-and-narrow I would still be a scientist and might still make a contribution to science. This broadminded scientific attitude (that is, how you go about it, not why, or whatever it may be one picks on to study) seemed very genial and straightforward to me until I suddenly realized through the following episode that it could never be that simple.

As a teaching aid in our anatomy course, Hamilton had us shown films of prolonged X-rays of the body, showing joint movements, and movements of the digestive tracts, peristalsis, etc. They were unique. Hopefully they still are. For exposure of the body to such prolonged X-rays produces massive X-ray burns and tissue devastation, and an agonizing death unless the human experimental animal is promptly put out of its misery. These were Nazi films of experiments done to Jews, purloined by the British at the end of World War II and now being used as teaching material.

It took a little while for what was going on to sink in. I saw one showing. I walked out with a friend of mine, John Owens. The other 200 or so students remained to sit and watch with apparent interest. We were sickened and outraged. We went to Professor Hamilton and expostulated with him. 'We are watching people being burned to death! How can you use this as teaching material?'

'Yes, I know. I agree with you. But it is unique teaching material. If we don't use it now, their deaths will have been in vain.'

Most of the students agreed with him. There was no 'movement' to boycott or ban these films. They were interesting. Just to indulge that interest (to hell with the 'interests' of 'science') for one second, made me feel I had caught the plague.

This incident intensified my terror of human beings, terror at the films themselves, at the minds behind the making of them, at the minds behind the bureaucratic and scientific efficiency that sustained with such blandness and blindness towards evil the social machinery of their distribution as well as of their making.

How had we all become so docile? Why did we take so much for granted? Why did most of us seem to believe what we were told by those we believed, and almost nothing else? *How* were we such conditioned creatures?

At this time I became very interested in hypnosis. Several of us formed a group to study hypnosis in theory and practice. We met every other week for some years. We hypnotized each other and anyone who allowed themselves to be used for practice. I was soon able to induce the usual trance phenomenon in the standard ways and used hypnosis in therapy with patients in my first postgraduate years in the Army and at Glasgow.

On one occasion a seasoned, proficient, professional hypnotist put me into a trance in front of several dozen people at a demonstration in his house. He asked me to choose a taste to taste. I chose a dry sherry. He gave me a dry sherry to savour, to roll around over and under my tongue and swallow at leisure. A very nice dry sherry. When I came out of trance, he invited me to try the sherry again. Its smell and taste were so repulsive that I could barely get it past my lips. He had a mouthwash in readiness which I clutched for desperately. Yes, it was the same drink, the foulest-tasting harmless concoction he could get a pharmacist to make up.

How could one's sense of *taste*, such an intimate sense, be so readily deceived? I could not believe my *taste*! This was not merely interesting. It was profoundly disquieting. It baffled me. It *scared* me. Under hypnosis one can reverse the sign of a stimulus in every sense-modality. The same hypnotist induced me to believe I saw only six people in a room filled with over sixty. I could induce a blister in someone who believed I was burning him when I was not and no tissue reaction when I was. And so on. Such phenomena of hypnotism are well documented and it is still unknown how far they go, for instance in the field of telepathic hypnotism. This being so, of what sort of texture was our everyday 'sense of reality'? What is the *real* taste of anything? In what sense are any phenomena really real? The whole issue of our whole sense of reality is called into question. Could the formally, explicitly induced, hypnotic trance be but one critical and fascinating instance of a much broader set of phenomena? The puzzles, possibilities and possible implications of hypnotism grabbed me then and have never let me go.

Seeing, we say, is believing. To what extent do we both believe what we see and see what we believe? How far does it go? How far is the whole feeling and fabric of our ordinary, everyday world socially programmed, an induced fiction, in which we are all enmeshed, except a few whose conditioning has not 'taken', or has broken down, or who have awakened from the spell – a motley crew of geniuses, psychotics and sages? If a foul concoction could taste like an excellent sherry, how do I know what a nice dry sherry 'really' tastes like, or anything else?

The few minutes of that particular hypnotic experiment deepened my sense of the mystery of the correlations between physical stimuli and our experience of them, of the embeddedness of sensation in mental set and setting, of the power of social dynamics and structure, of our personal bonds and bondage to influence, even to determine our beliefs, thoughts, sensations, perceptions, feelings, constructions and conduct to an indeterminable extent.

Our personal 'reality', I realized, is a very dependent variable, the outcome or product of factors that do not seem to depend on this 'reality', but to exist in some independent 'reality' which affects us but is beyond us.

'We' may be even more the stuff that dreams are made on than we can imagine even our dreams to be made on.

We have to distinguish a formally set-up hypnotic session, as a set-piece in the laboratory, in the consulting room or on stage, from the sort of thing that happens in ordinary life, usually without anyone involved knowing what is happening. Hypnosis in the restricted formal sense is a special case of *induction*. It is one of the wide variety of ways we induce others to see, hear, touch, smell, believe, think, feel, desire, and do whatever we want them to. Hypnosis seemed to offer an extraordinarily simple (if one got the hang of it) way to play around with manipulation, scientific exploration, techniques of interpersonal induction – that is, of *power* – in the domain where people transact with people and we try to induce others to do and be what we want and vice versa. Techniques of interpersonal manipulation, control and power do not seem to induce the unhappy to be happy, the depressed to be cheerful, the frantic to be calm, the disorientated to be orientated, the confused to be clear, the deluded to drop their unacceptable beliefs and adopt acceptable ones. Those with the most unacceptable beliefs are often most resistant to attempts to change them. They are notoriously 'inaccessible' to personal and environmental manipulation. They can still be got at via the brain by psychotropic (mind-changing) chemicals.

Remember the 'induction' of Winston Smith in *Nineteen Eighty-Four* in which O'Brien forces Winston to believe that he sees five fingers instead of four. When Orwell wrote that, in 1948, Milton Erickson was already putting that sort of manipulation into practice, as recounted by Jay Haley:

> I recall a demonstration Erickson once did before a large audience. He asked for a volunteer, and a young man came up and sat down with him. Erickson's only trance induction was to ask the young man to put his hands on his knees. Then he said, 'Would you be willing to continue to see your hands on your knees?' The young man said he would. While talking with him, Erickson gestured to a colleague on the other side of the young man, and the colleague lifted up the young man's arm and it remained in the air. Erickson said to the young man, 'How many hands do you have?' 'Two, of course,' said the young man. 'I'd like you to count them as I point to them,' said Erickson. 'All right,' said the young man, in a rather patronizing way. Erickson pointed to the hand on one knee. The young man said, 'One.' Erickson pointed to the vacant other knee, where the young man had agreed to continue to see his hand, and the young man said, 'Two.' Then Erickson pointed to the hand up in the air. The young man stared at it, puzzled. 'How do you explain that other hand?' asked Erickson. 'I don't know,' said the young man. 'I guess I should be in a circus.' That hypnotic induction took about as long as it took me to describe it here.[4]

The puzzle turns in on itself. How can we tell when, or if, we might not be enveloped in a trance, a spell, an enchantment, a dream, some blindness we are blind to, an ignorance we ignore? How can one see into, see through, fathom or wake up, or be sure one is awake?

It is lonely and risky to lose one's common sense. The dogmatic dream that one is the *only* person who can see things as they are is usually taken as an index of an unsound mind. When I started to meet psychotic patients professionally, I found, to my alarm, that sometimes I could see their point of view only too well. If I did not wish to ruin my career, I would have to be very circumspect.

Are you willing to continue to see that right hand resting there on the arm of your chair? I am not giving you a suggestion or an order. I am just asking you an 'innocent' question for an innocent agreement. When many people agree to be 'married', they, in effect, agree to continue to see a 'marriage' there, even when it has long gone. Their 'marriage' has become, as it were, a sort of hallucination, the ghost of a lingering illusion. What other such agreements may we have made that we may have agreed to forget we made?

I investigated 'scientifically' revivalist meetings, séances, spiritualist meetings, anything paranormal. I timed my heart on a stopwatch, as it pounded and quickened at crunch moments in revivalist meetings. I exposed myself to Billy Graham. A great revivalist stage-craftsman like him could count on 'converting' about the same percentage (10 per cent) at a performance as a first-class hypnotist. At these revivalist meetings in Glasgow, my tongue could go dry, my throat ache, heart thump, palms sweat at appropriate dramatic moments in the telling of the Gospel to Sinners that they may repent by the Grace of the Lord.

I can still be affected. Is it all totally, economically, culturally, anthropologically conditioned? Is it all mumbojumbo? Is it a way of touching on profoundest truth?

I was not reconverted, but I did become convinced about the existence of paranormal happenings. At the same time, I realized that a sense of conviction does not arise, or need not arise, out of statistics, but out of one single 'convincing' moment.

One such moment for me was an occasion on which a friend and I went to a crowded spiritualist meeting in a strange part of Glasgow. Neither of us knew anyone there;

as far as we knew no one knew us. We slipped in quietly by
the back door. We could not see the medium, nor she us, in
the dim light, across a room filled with over fifty people.
She interrupted what she was on about to say that two
young men had entered. They were welcome. They were
medical students. One of them came from Gourock (him).
One of them had an aunt called Mysie (me). The one who
came from Gourock had an address book in his left-hand
pocket (he had) in which, if he now got it out, opened it and
looked at it (he did) he would be looking at a certain
telephone number (that was the number he was looking at).

The first surgical operation I attended, at the Glasgow
Royal Infirmary, was very atypical of hospital surgery in this
day and age. It was a mid-thigh amputation on an old,
seasoned and pickled sea-salt who was beginning to develop gangrene due to advanced arteriosclerosis. His heart
and lungs were not in good shape. It was thought he would
not stand a chance with a general anaesthetic, so it was
decided to try out a procedure that had been reported from
Australia: ice-pack anaesthesia. The surgeon ordered his
left leg, which was the one to be amputated, to be packed in
ice the night before and for him to be given a bottle of
whisky before the night-staff went off. The operation was to
be performed first thing in the morning.

At the first cut of the knife he went wild, screaming,
yelling and cursing. It was evident that the ice-pack had not
had its desired effect and, it turned out, the nurse on night-
duty who had given him a bottle of whisky had no idea of
what a bottle of whisky meant in the real world and had
given him the contents of a four-ounce hospital bottle,
which he had downed in one gulp. It did not touch him at
all.

Anyway, it was too late to turn back. He had to be held
down and I saw an old-style amputation. The whole thing.

However shocking such things are, I could 'take' them.
Life has to go on. Every gamble does not come off. It is no

one's fault really. The next patient is already on the table. There is no time to cry over spilt blood. But there were other sorts of suffering that went beyond all reason and struck terror right into my bone-marrow.

In the same surgery ward there was a man in his forties, with what was then called *myositis ossificans progressiva* (*fibro dysplasia ossificans*), a condition in which muscles turn to bone.

It is a disease of great rarity. He sat in his chair utterly expressionless. His eyes could move strictly horizontally from left to right. No other voluntary movement seemed possible. His rib-cage was fixed. His tongue could not move. He was tube-fed. His diaphragm still moved slightly. He was almost completely turned to bone. He died of asphyxiation very gradually, over weeks, as finally his diaphragm turned to bone.

I was horrified and terrified. It was a genetic condition. It could not be put down to human error, in any obvious way to human evil. These terrible diseases I saw turned me totally against any God who was supposed to be omnipotent and good. If He were omnipotent how could He be good if He were responsible for the creation of such suffering? I could tell myself that only through the very spirit of love, our Holy Spirit, or in John Wycliffe's translation our Healthy Spirit, God incarnate in us, could I feel such outrage. Maybe God couldn't help it. But then how could He be omnipotent? I told myself that this was all human reasoning: that God, if He existed, must be infinitely beyond the paltry projections of my idealized conception of my own ideals. I was terrified of Him if He existed, and terrified if He did not. Life was a ghastly joke. We were the joke, but I could not see it. Or else it signified nothing. I could not forget, or go beyond, the conflict. And it would not somehow or other melt away.

At the end of our first year as medical students, we paid a traditional visit to the Royal Gartnavel Mental Hospital, Glasgow.

This was the first time I had been in a mental hospital. Over a hundred students assembled in the main hall and the Superintendent, Dr Angus MacNiven, from a stage platform, gave a short talk about the hospital and psychiatry and introduced and talked with four or five patients. These were the first psychiatric patients I had ever set eyes upon.

I came in late. There were two men on the stage sitting on chairs, having a chat. One of them, in impeccable dress, with a cheerful flower in his buttonhole, sat with composure and assurance, talked fluently with the other man, who had his legs twisted around each other, grimaced, stammered, fidgeted, all but picked his nose, and wriggled around in his chair.

It was not until that interview ended, when the patient got up, gave a bow and left the stage that I realized that Dr MacNiven was the man I had taken to be the patient. Years later, after medical school, six months in a neurosurgical unit and two years as a psychiatrist in the British Army, he was very amused when, now a registrar on his staff, I told him the story.

This was a very decent interview. It sounded like two old friends chatting about the hospital, the changes they had seen. The patient had been in the hospital longer than MacNiven, had been there in the time of D. K. Henderson, later Professor of Psychiatry at Edinburgh University and co-author with Gillespie of a book that became a standard text in British psychiatry.[5] The patient claimed to have been mentioned in despatches, as it were, in that book for calling D. K. Henderson 'the Kaiser', which was cited as an example of a paranoid delusion.

After a lifetime of social catastrophes in states of manic excitement he had settled into a room in Gentlemen's West Wing, the paying part of the hospital, where most of the time he lived quietly in a state of indefatigable good humour.

In a sense, my first patient was my father. In my last year at school he had what is called a 'nervous breakdown', and was laid off work for three months. He had started to tremble, inexplicably. Nothing like it had ever overtaken him before. For most of the three months he lay in bed. Without any drugs. I sat beside him for some time every day. Our family doctor looked in on him occasionally to see that he was all right.

He was troubled in mind. Thinking about that time now, I imagine that his experiences in World War I, the Tank Corps in Africa, the Royal Air Corps, must have had a lot to do with it, and his unhappy life with my mother . . . but he never ever talked to me about what 'the war' meant to him personally, and, I imagine, he had too great a sense of propriety and loyalty to her to talk to me about that sort of thing.

But he did go on about his relations with his colleagues in his job on 'the Mains' (the network of electric cables that runs under the ground in cities) and I had heard some things before about his relations with his father.

His boss, his immediate superior, was about to retire. My father was due to step into his shoes, if all went as usual. But he suspected that his chief would stop his 'promotion'. His chief was a Christian Scientist, who did not believe in evil. My father thought that Inglis did not want him to succeed him (Inglis) because he (Inglis) thought he (my father) was an atheist.

As I have indicated, this was a very serious and touchy subject – I myself had accused my father vehemently of being an atheist. Atheist or not (and I never thought he was more of an atheist than Albert Schweitzer or Paul Tillich), my father was one of the purest spirits I have ever come across. Except for his father, I had never heard him hold anything against anyone. But I don't think he ever forgave his father for, as he believed, having done in his mother by turning her into 'a nervous wreck'. When my father and I were walking away from Old Pa's grave at his funeral, my father turned to me and said, 'Now the bastard's dead.' They were his only words.

I told my father that I thought it was very unlikely that his chief Inglis was trying to do him in. Even if he was, I could not imagine that my father was going on trembling just at the possibility of not getting a promotion, however important that undoubtedly was. It was Old Pa, his father, it must be all about. Inglis was not Old Pa. Nor could I buy the atheist issue. It was Old Pa again. Old Pa in the sky.

The 'nervous breakdown' lasted under three months. For whatever reasons, it came on; for whatever reasons, it passed. He went back to work, resumed his position as Principal Baritone at the Glasgow University Chapel Choir and, shortly, on Inglis's retirement, he got Inglis's job, retained it and moved on to another promotion before his own retirement.

He later told me that what I had said to him about Inglis and God and Old Pa counted for ninety-five per cent of his recovery.

My remarks to my father, I later discovered, would be called 'interpretations'. I had no idea at the time that I was making 'interpretations' of a father-transference from Old Pa to God and the boss.

In subsequent years I would get waves of trepidation at the thought of 'taking after' Old Pa. Of 'turning out like' Old Pa. Putting it in technical psychoanalytic language, I think now that I missed then that he was projecting Old Pa on to me. In those three months we switched positions from son to father to son. I became in a sense his father. But his projection, his father-transference on to me, passed unbeknown to either of us. The transaction was unconscious and some sort of projection of his father on to me (a good father as well as a bad father) took place in me then with reverberating, very ambiguous effects through the years to the present.

Something overtook my father's father when he was in his fifties and my father was a youth. Something overtook my father when he was in his fifties and I was a youth. I am in my fifties and I have a son who is a youth. I feel rocked by waves of hundreds of years.

My father spent the last ten years of his life confined in a psychogeriatric unit.

One day he had stumbled, fallen and cracked his head. No fractures, but his memory had gone. Some time after that he got up one morning, put on his homburg hat, took his rolled umbrella and went out for a walk. Unfortunately, he had forgotten to put his clothes on. He had to be put away, in a 'closed' ward. He would be let out to donner around the grounds, sit on a bench and have a cup of tea in the cafeteria. He donnered out of the grounds two or three times in those last ten years, got lost and had to be brought back by the police. Once he went to a police station, and announced, 'I am an old gentleman and I have lost his way.' He did not know his name or where he came from or where he was or anything about his life. Latterly he had to be helped to dress and undress. He could blow his own nose, wipe his own mouth, eat, get in and out of bed by himself and do most things for himself but was 'too much' for my mother, already a frail old lady. Besides she could not keep him locked up, and it was out of the question for him to go out on the street in his state. In hospital (Leverndale, Glasgow), he was treated very warmly, considerately and respectfully by the staff. During the whole ten years nothing in the way they treated my Dad rubbed me the wrong way. He was no exception. I know that psychiatric institutions need not be inhumane.

My first encounter with real psychiatric patients was in the wards of the Psychiatric Unit in Duke Street Hospital, Glasgow, where I attended my first clinical classes in psychiatry under the consultant there, Dr Sclare, whose son was to follow in his father's footsteps and become a distinguished psychiatrist.

One of the patients in the ward was a thin, middle-aged

man with a wife and family, who was, I think, a clerk. The nuclear problems of psychiatry, which confront all psychiatrists day in and day out, which nag anyone who thinks about them, are all in this one case. There is nothing especially unusual about it. That is why it is so interesting. It is so typical. What is, I think, today very unusual was that I actually saw someone going into a state of catatonic immobility over a period of two weeks. Very few psychiatrists must ever witness that now because the process would be stopped or transformed by drugs and electric shocks if he were admitted in time. I do not know what became of him.

He had no complaints. He said nothing. He was in hospital at his wife's instigation. As far as was known, until 'this' started to happen he had been a normal person living a normal life. For no known reason, about two months earlier, he started not to do things. He would stand in front of the mirror and not tie his tie. If his wife prodded him, he would do it. Then, if she started it, he would finish it. But it had got beyond her and now he was in a bed in a psychiatric unit.

He might sit up, or he might have to be sat up. He might stand up, or he might have to be stood. If he was started off, he would put his clothes on, then stand, or maybe take a few steps in some direction. There were all sorts of 'somethings' he would complete if started, then stop. These 'somethings' seemed to be the motions we go through in doing the things we have such names for as: getting out of bed, putting clothes on, urinating, unbuttoning and buttoning up, washing hands and face, shaving, brushing teeth, combing hair, walking, sitting down, lifting a cup, cutting a loaf of bread, buttering it, putting it in one's mouth, swallowing it. The units became smaller and smaller until he would hardly lift a finger to do anything for himself. The lazy bastard! He tried the patience of the nursing staff.

On physical examination nothing abnormal was detected.

It never is. No one had the faintest idea why he was carrying on like that. No one has now. He had nothing to say. He did not seem to be hallucinating. Impossible to tell really what sort of state of mind he was in. His eyes were alive. He blinked.

He was diagnosed first, descriptively, as a case of *abulia* (absence of will). *Abulia* could be hysterical or psychotic or malingering. Within a few weeks he could be presented as a typical catatonic.

Could I now pick out a catatonic's immobility from an actor's immobility mimicking catatonic immobility? Could I tell by looking and examining whether someone was in deep meditation, deep trance, under hypnosis, pretending to be paralysed, actually paralysed, frozen stiff with fear, or could in fact move but must not and does not? Someone who can't move and wants to, who can move and does not want to, someone who has forgotten how to, someone who is elsewhere, someone who is all there and not at all here, someone who thinks he can't but could if he thought he could. Is he a pillar of salt? Is he god incarnate stone? Is he the still centre of the turning world? Is something the matter with his neurochemistry?

I failed my final medical examinations completely first time.

I'll never know why I failed every subject in every way. I was simply told to repeat the whole affair next time and given no compulsory *courses* to retake. Most unusual. I've always wondered whether my failure might have had something to do with our Final Year Dinner, when, sitting with the professors at the top of the table, as an after-dinner speaker, I drank too much whisky, claret and port, and expressed far too candidly what I felt about a few things in medicine.

I filled in the next six months until I could take them again as a full-time, half-paid, unqualified internist, living in at the Psychiatric Unit at Stobhill Hospital in Glasgow.

As well as being the usual sort of psychiatric unit in a general hospital, it housed about eighty men and women who had caught what was thought to be the 'flu in 1927, but it turned out to be *encephalitis lethargica*. They were the devastated survivors of an epidemic that swept Europe then. It started off just like the 'flu, but it was an inflammation of the brain that either struck one dead or caused one to linger on for years demented, drooling, contorted and paralysed.

There can be no doubt. These people's central nervous systems were physically, organically devastated by the ravages of a viral infection of the brain. Damage must be deeply organic, structural, and something was wrong with their molecular-cellular metabolism, still to be finally unravelled. It is a terrifying condition to see. And at the same time the psychiatric wards were full of the usual assortment of mentally ill people, who all had nothing physically the matter with them as far as one could tell, but – 'it *must* be organic'.

I now knew what I wanted to go for. Neurology, neuropsychiatry, psychiatry, not forgetting hypnosis.

NEUROSURGERY

I became completely focused on the central nervous system. How does the brain produce the mind? Or is it the other way round? Or are both questions so stupid they should be dropped immediately? If I 'went in for' neurology I would have a chance of becoming clinically scientific about an area I could not stop thinking about, and even agonizing over, very unscientifically. So when I graduated, rather impetuously and recklessly from the point of view of the prudent cultivation of a balanced orthodox medical career, I took a job that was going as an internist in a neurosurgical unit, skipping the usual two postgraduate years of internships in general medicine and surgery.

The Glasgow and Western Scotland Neurosurgical Unit

was situated at Killearn, not far from Loch Lomond, in one of the most beautiful parts of the world, comparable at its sweetest and most delicately lyrical to Kashmir. Then, as now, there were many weekend motorists and motor-cyclists. Saturday afternoons, when the pubs used to close for a few hours, we would not be surprised to get in two or three characters with their brains oozing out from the bonnie bonnie banks of Loch Lomond.

As a student I had been up and down that winding road on the west bank of Loch Lomond full of Guinness and whisky at 80 m.p.h. many times in the middle of winter, in all sorts of weather.

Two of my closest friends died on that road. But it was not until I saw those bashed-in skulls and seeping brains, and, if not death itself, then its after-effects, that I really lost my taste for drunken motorcycle driving – usually without a helmet in those days. Those were also the days before breathalyzers. Terror struck into my bones again. The awful disabilities that could be the outcome of a successful operation. A life was saved, with bits and pieces of brain left.

My mind would play back in slow motion how we went round that blind corner, blind drunk: waves of remorse, relief, panic I had never felt at the time; shame, at the risks we took with other people's lives; more waves and pangs, panic, panic. Utter madness!

The unit also received the whole range of a neurosurgical and neurological unit, from cerebellar abscesses to low back-pain.

My tasks were to do general systemic and neurological examinations, assist at operations, accompany consultants on ward rounds; above all, to get needles into veins for drawing off blood, to set up 'drips' without thrombosing the patients' arms, to do lumbar punctures without turning the lower back into a pincushion, and to get a canula through a burr-hole (a hole made in the skull by the surgeon) to draw off cerebral spinal fluid from the lateral ventricle without turning the temporal lobe into mush. Unfortunately and unavoidably, these basic skills can only be acquired by practice.

All the patients had something very definitely the matter with their central nervous systems. One of my tasks was to attend to people who were unconscious, in deep coma. Several 'brain-dead' people were 'routinely' kept alive. 'They' were little more than 'heart-lung preparations'. They were kept going mainly as a technical exercise. I don't think any new scientific knowledge came out of it. Neurosurgical units around the world were keeping other brain-dead people alive and there was a competition going on on the world grapevine as to who could keep what sort of post-traumatic or post-operative brain-damaged human organism going longest. We thought we held one record for a type of mid-brain injury, until we learned that a body as brainless as ours was still going strong after two years in a neurosurgical unit in Japan. Such callousness did not obliterate concern. They co-existed.

The practice I got at that time in 'finding' a vein when all veins had 'collapsed', getting the needle into it and something to flow through the needle probably saved several lives, a year later, at the British Army's deep insulin unit at Netley, near Southampton, when 'deep' insulin 'death' comas were in vogue.

There were three neurosurgical chiefs at the unit: Paterson, Robertson and Schorstein. There was a 'lobotomy controversy' going on. Paterson and Schorstein refused to do lobotomies. Robertson did them, at the behest of Dr MacNiven. I was assigned to assist Paterson and Schorstein.

Paterson was small, wiry, fit, approaching the end of his serious surgical career, still doing operations of over six hours at a stretch. My job in the surgical theatre consisted of little else than holding forceps out of the way and applying a light (from a movable torch attached to my forehead) to the site of the operation. The most exacting thing was to keep the beam steadily on focus in the surgical area deep in the brain. It required one to bend one's shoulders, crane one's neck forward, keep it completely immobile, masked, totally covered in sterile clothing, crown of the head to soles of the feet; intolerable pain in one's neck and back, concentration, exhaustion . . . I passed out twice. At least I managed to collapse sideways and backwards.

It was no disgrace. Paterson did not hold it against me but assured me that I had no instinct for brain surgery. He encouraged me in my neurological ambitions, however. Though not my metaphysical speculations. He had no time for any neurological theories or armchair speculations which were not practical and pragmatic when it came to the crunch. Like some other brain surgeons he did try to conceal a sense of superiority over 'mere' neurologists. As a neurosurgeon he was every bit a neurologist and had the daily experience of actually operating on brains in all sorts of conditions into the bargain. A psychiatrist who was not even a competent neurologist was really beyond the pale as far as he was concerned. He could not be taken as a clinical equal. Clinically, neurosurgeons are entitled to that sense of authority that comes from physical intimacy with the human brain and nervous system, steeped as they are – day in, day out, year in, year out – in observing correlations between brain damage and disease, and loss of function and partial or complete recovery of function.

We internists just seemed to be 'at it' all the time. Work and sleep. A neurosurgical unit is no place for armchair speculation. I had never been so physically 'stretched' before. And through it all, I was in more mental and even physical torture than ever before over all the problems that baffled me day and night.

At three o'clock in the morning in the changing room after one operating session that had been going for hours, Joe Schorstein decided to check me out. He proceeded to grill me from Heraclitus and, in between, Kant, Hegel, Nietzsche, Husserl, Heidegger, in very specific detail. The interrogation went on for over two hours before Joe was 'convinced'. Then began a real argument that went on for another two hours. No one, before or since, has put me through such a grinder.

After that night Joe adopted me as his pupil; he became my spiritual father, neurological and intellectual mentor, and guide to European literature.

Joe Schorstein FRCS was eighteen years older than I was. He was the son of a Hasidic Rabbi in a village some miles from Vienna. He had a deeply lined face that made him look older than he was, and was small and stocky; from somewhere he got his stamina. His father was also imbued with European culture and had a PhD in philosophy from Heidelberg. When Joe was ten, his father punished him for something by having him study Kant's *Critique of Pure Reason* for three months. Then he had to stand in front of his father in his study and satisfy him under interrogation that he had assimilated it properly.

At the age of sixteen, Joe became converted to communism. His father disowned him. He went to Prague; began medical training there; fled to London when the going was still good; graduated there; studied under Sir Jeffrey Jefferson in Manchester; went into the British Army as a neurosurgeon, became chief of the No. 1 Neurosurgical Unit to the British Army from El Alamein through Africa and Italy to Austria at the end of the war. In 1951 he was forty-one, one of the triumvirate of senior neurosurgeons at the Glasgow and West of Scotland Neurosurgical Unit. His speciality was casualty surgery, but he did the whole range. He was in the right place in this territory.

He had had plenty of practice – eighteen hours a day for spells, he said, from El Alamein to Austria. He was a brilliant technician and an accomplished neurologist and one of the most tormented human beings I have ever met.

He was the first older, fully educated European intellectual I had come to know. He seemed to be the incarnation of all the positions of the European consciousness: Hasidism, Marxism, science and nihilism. He believed in the

Crucifixion, but could not believe in the Resurrection. And the Crucifixion without the Resurrection is the ultimate cosmic nightmare. He could not sleep. He could not awake from that nightmare. He had, to varying degrees, knowledge of Greek, Latin, Hebrew, Czech, French, Italian, English, German, and for all I know bits of Portuguese and Bulgarian too.

He was very alone and lonely, married with three children.

'Nietzsche,' he would say, 'may not have been a better philosopher than Descartes, but he was a far more desperate man.' No one who had not given up 'dirty' hope could possibly be relevant now. The old *Titanic* was already sinking. Some were playing cards. He had met Jaspers, Heidegger and Buber. He was my first personal link with 'the greats'. He had walked out of a lecture by Alfred Adler. He was a master of the European tradition to which I was beginning to be mature enough to presume to belong.

He was also very cultivated musically. He sang Hasidic and Central European songs, many of which I first heard from him. I can still surprise a Central European Jew by coming out with one of them. 'How did you come across *that* one?!'

It is a great pity that Schorstein hardly wrote anything down about his Hasidic, theological and philosophical reflections. He meditated, prayed, thought, and spoke to a few. He spoke as he might have written, and, in the only paper I know of in which he committed that sort of thing to writing, he wrote as he was speaking during all the time I knew him.[6]

I learned in my brief spell in this neurosurgical unit how difficult it is, for me at least, to keep an open heart to the suffering and at the same time to remain efficient, to be able to move on to the next patient and to put out of one's mind the last.

> He was ten years of age and had *hydrocephalus* due to
> an inoperable tumour the size of a very small pea, just
> at the right place to stop his cerebrospinal fluid from

getting out of his head: which is to say that he had
water on the brain and it was bursting his head, so
that the brain was becoming stretched out into a
thinning rim, and his skull bones likewise. He was in
excruciating and unremitting pain.

One of my jobs was to put a long needle into this
ever-increasing fluid to let it out. I had to do this
twice a day and the so-clear fluid that was killing him
would leap out at me from his massive ten-year-old
head, rising in a brief column to several feet,
sometimes hitting my face. . . . But this little boy
unmistakably endured agony. He would quietly cry in
pain. If he could only have shrieked or complained.
. . . And he knew he was going to die.

He had started reading *The Pickwick Papers*. The
one thing he asked God for, he told me, was that he
be allowed to finish this book before he died.

He died before it was half finished.*

She was nineteen, and a circus-horse rider. She and her
horse fell. The horse rolled over her head and had to be
destroyed. She was completely 'out' for several days. When
she came round, she *was* a horse. She looked like a horse. She
had horse's eyes. She neighed. She grazed on the grass
outside the ward, naked, on all fours. After three or four
weeks she turned into herself again, over the course of two or
three days. I wanted *desperately* to *understand* this sort of thing.

There was a passage from Thomas Traherne (somewhat
changed from the original) I kept repeating to myself. This
is how I remember remembering it:

He knows nothing as he ought to know, unless he knows
its relations to God, angels and men, time and eternity.

To keep sight of that, while studying the Babinski Reflex
clinically, was agonizing; the skull seemed at times the
Golgotha of the spirit.

* R. D. Laing, *The Bird of Paradise*, Penguin, 1967, p. 146.

FOUR

The Army

1951 was the time of the Korean war, and in the UK a time of universal conscription for military service for a minimum of two years. I was exempted from military service because of asthma.

I corresponded with Karl Jaspers, the Swiss psychiatrist-philosopher. He agreed to 'take me on' once a week to begin with, and to arrange for me to attend the Neuro-psychiatric Department at the University of Basel under his friend, Professor Stachelin. I was given a scholarship through Glasgow University to study with him in Basel. Then the British Army extended their dragnet to include my medical grade. I went before a board in Edinburgh who determined that I would serve 'the cause' better by putting in two years in the British Army than in Basel with Jaspers. The crunch in the minds of the members of the board seemed to be that, although Jaspers had written and kept up to date one of the fundamental textbooks on psychiatry,[7] he had not practised psychiatry for many years. He was now 'just' a philosopher. I was honoured that they were pre-pared to jump me up two years in advance of my expected clinical status.

Everyone said, 'But, Dr Laing, Jaspers is just armchair now, isn't he?' It would be better for my clinical career to go into the Army. I could have my choice, neurology or psychiatry, although I had had only six months' postgrad-uate experience. Both neurology and psychiatry in the British Army had a good, wide reputation. I chose psy-chiatry. Schorstein thought I was making a big mistake. They did not want me to 'throw away the best "clinical" years of my life', by getting diverted into armchair philosophy. Maybe they were right, but at the time I thought they were being shortsighted.

When I entered the British Army, my mind was in a theoretical ferment: historical materialism, nihilism, theology, philosophy, psychology, neurology; the discovery of phenomenology; Heidegger, Sartre, Merleau-Ponty, Husserl; the discovery of the distinctions between understanding and explanation; the translation of the hermeneutics of the text to the hermeneutics of interpersonal relations; the twin figures, for me, of Kierkegaard and Nietzsche, Christ and Anti-Christ, the knight of faith, the destiny of nihilism; Nietzsche's critique of 'convictions' and his disposal of the ego, free will, and the problems of psychiatry and psychopathology; Heidegger and the question of being, what is to be? Wittgenstein: the destruction of that question. Nietzsche and Wittgenstein: history. The socio-economic material reality of society. The British Army. The Korean war. The Bomb.

I had given up an active commitment to politics in the usual sense of the term as a student, not out of any matter of principle, but regretfully, because I felt I was not 'cut out for it' – and there was another branch of politics into which I began to want to look more closely – our person-to-person politics that permeate all socio-economic, intra- or inter-class, national or racial relations. The politics of the basic human bond itself. The politics of love. I saw love as crucified. But I could not see its resurrection. That was my nightmare. And yet the betrayal of love is one's entry into the pure lands of nihilism.

In our first weeks of induction into the Royal Army Medical Corps we were located at a hospital on the Thames Embankment and then at one near Aldershot.

At that time we were told a few things in the course of the lectures we attended. I have no idea whether they were true or not, but they effectively changed my attitude to the Bomb.

Biochemical warfare. Germ warfare, chemical agents, viruses, nerve gases.

'Everyone' had been very surprised that World War II had ended without any of that stuff being tried out. Maybe in some quarters there was a measure of disappointment as well as relief. Why had Hitler not tossed a few canisters of super-plague virus over Russia, Britain, North America, as a last fling when he had the stuff? The British and American Armies, by courtesy of the *Wehrmacht*, so the story went, got to vast vats of plague viruses twenty times or more (who knows?) virulent than ordinary plague. That at least was something. *We* got hold of all that, not the Russians. But God knows what the Russians had up their sleeves.

In the next war (as I said, no one ever thought that the last one was the last one) all that sort of stuff would have to be brought out. Of course it meant wiping out most or all of our own population, but that would happen anyway. The important point was that we would take the enemy with us and they knew that.

The central British Army Psychiatric Unit at Netley contained an insulin unit of about twenty beds, and neurotic and psychotic divisions.

Insulin was administered at six o'clock in the morning and within four hours the patients began to go into coma. The course of insulin started off with ten units, increased daily by ten units until the patients went into deep comas and sometimes epileptic fits. The policy was to put it in at a level at which epileptic fits were liable to occur, but to avoid them if possible. Backs could break. Light is extremely epileptogenic under a lot of insulin. The ward was entirely blacked out. When people started to go into coma we, the staff, moved around in total darkness, penetrated only by the rays of the torches on hinges we had strapped to our foreheads. It was essential to get each patient out of his or her coma before too long, because if we did not, the coma became 'irreversible'. Around ten o'clock, we poured quantities of 50 per cent glucose into the patients through stomach tubes. We hoped we had got the tube into the stomach rather than the lungs. Difficult to tell sometimes with someone in a coma. We often had to put up pressurized glucose drips in the darkness for patients already completely collapsed whose veins had disappeared. There were those who 'had no veins left' because of thrombosis everywhere caused by veins bursting under pressure, and needles would 'miss the vein', glucose solution pouring into the tissues. One might have to take a scalpel to 'cut down' and stick a needle into something one just hoped was not an artery or a nerve. We had only our headlights.

Since 'tube-feeds', 'veins' and 'drips', and surgical headlights were the order of the day, I had an ideal training in my brief but intense six months' neurosurgical job.

After some weeks I was sent up to meet Dr Mayer-Gross, one of the world's authorities on insulin-coma treatment, whose insulin unit at Dumfries in Scotland was world famous. Joe Schorstein had been his patient. The Army wanted him to vet me for the insulin unit and for him to pass on any tips he could in a short visit.

Mayer-Gross had the curtains drawn, the ward in a soft light, not pitch darkness. The atmosphere he exuded was warm and embracing. But the British Army patients were escalated through insulin and plunged deeply into coma faster than the patients he was treating, so were more liable to have major epileptic seizures, which, once started, are very difficult to control.

I had seen more epileptic fits than usual for someone of my clinical age, in both the post-encephalitic Parkinsonian unit at Stobhill and at the neurosurgical and neurological unit at Killearn. The aura, the cry, the fall and the fit. The tonus, the conus, the piss and the shit. It never looks pleasant. I had sat and watched a boy of ten die through a series of marching epileptic fits – a twitch in the thumb spreads out and 'marches' rapidly and inexorably throughout the muscles of the body. I hated epileptic fits. But there was an idea in the air, propounded in particular by Ugo

Cerletti, Professor of Psychiatry at Rome University, that epileptic fits might be good for schizophrenia. Cerletti was credited with designing the snow-camouflage equipment for the Italian Army in World War I. One of his special interests was electricity and the brain. He had described how one day in a slaughter-house he saw the way pigs were slaughtered, first being stunned on the head with an electric shock, then their throats being slit. It occurred to him that if *that* amount of electricity could not even kill a pig, then the way was open to apply electricity to the brains of human beings and no better way to start a new chapter of science than with the brains of schizophrenics.

Cerletti believed that schizophrenia and epilepsy bore some sort of inverse relation to each other. Schizophrenic epileptics seemed less schizophrenic after an epileptic fit. Therefore, how about giving schizophrenics epilepsy or, less crudely, giving schizophrenics an electric cerebral lavage, or shower? It might clean out or wash up their clogged up or dirty brains. Hence *electric* shocks could induce epilepsy and muscle relaxants could prevent an actual seizure recurring.*

The idea of 'death comas' was also in the air – the death and rebirth archetype, taken literally. In deep insulin coma the patient comes very close to real physical death and sometimes actually dies. Some people feel they do die, and they may in fact do so. They certainly look as though they have. Breathing, pulse, heartbeat may be imperceptible for long seconds, maybe minutes.

Might not this dip into death be therapeutic? The brain is chemically poisoned in some way and the mind is full of unintelligible gibberish. Wash it out, wipe it, clean the brain

* This account is based mainly on several of Cerletti's papers; the gist of all of them is in a paper I reproduced *in toto* in my book *The Facts of Life*. The constructions not in Cerletti's paper are, I hope, a fair account of the word-of-mouth psychiatric conventional fabric of the time.

and cleanse the mind: how about a fresh start, a new beginning, a rebirth, a resurrection? Mayer-Gross preferred to give less insulin and induce the epilepsy in a more controlled way, by electric shocks in the middle of the coma.

Through the year I was in this Army psychiatric unit, the staff in the psychotic wing had strict orders not to talk to the patients or to encourage the patients to talk to them, or to each other, or to themselves, or at all. No patient was expected to speak to a member of staff unless spoken to. Talking between patients was observed, reported and broken up. Pairing off was prevented. Friendship was not forbidden because psychotics are incapable of it. But they might form a *folie à deux*: difficult to destroy clinically, but still clinically interesting if the worst came to the worst.

You must not let a schizophrenic talk to you. It aggravates the psychotic process. It is like promoting a haemorrhage in a haemophiliac or giving a laxative to someone with diarrhoea. It inflames the brain and fans the psychosis. As in bone fractures, so with fractured minds: *immobilization* is the answer. No communication is better than any for the period of treatment.

As a lieutenant expected to enforce these commands, I was of course not subject to them myself. I did mental examinations as well as physical examinations. Take seven from a hundred. What is the meaning of 'People in glass houses should not throw stones'? Name, rank, number, age, married or single, name of the prime minister, the day of the week, the month of the year, the year, who was Jesus Christ? Since 'Jesus fuckin' Christ' is such a common Army expression, I tried out this last question in an informal survey on a random sample of several dozen non-commissioned ranks and found that, without its having any statistical significance, over 10 per cent had not the slightest idea what the term or the expression meant.

As an officer and a psychiatrist, I asked the patients on

insulin about their hallucinations and delusions. One of them had the interesting delusion that he was humped out of bed in his drugged sleep in the middle of the night, dragged out of the ward and beaten up somewhere by two men in Army uniforms. Another patient came up with the same delusion. An interesting case of communication without words: telepathic *folie à deux*. Then a third patient came up with the same delusion: *folie à trois*. Then a fourth: *folie à quatre* . . . ? It suddenly occurred to me . . . maybe? Eventually, it blew out into a court-martial. A corporal and private on night duty were court-martialled, convicted, and given a dishonourable discharge with two years' hard labour.*

Most of my time was spent in a neurotic–psychopathic–alcoholic-battle–neurosis–anything-goes–miscellaneous ward.

There were pre-tranquillizer drugs – barbiturates, chloralhydrate, paraldehyde, electric shocks, 'modified' insulin, straitjackets, 'padded cells', injections, tube-feeds, amytal abreactions, antibuse, hypnosis.

The Army espoused vigorous, 'muscular' treatment for its psychiatric casualties and patients. It 'looked after its own' by giving them the benefit of as active a treatment as was going in 'the best' civilian centres. Even an officer could go psychotic. You could not hold it against him any more than you could cancer.

* After having written this very paragraph I started to wonder – could I be making this up? The phone rang. A man at the other end said, 'Is that Dr Laing?' 'Yes.' He went on to say that his father had just been telling him of what it had been like in Netley for him as a patient – a private in the Army, diagnosed schizophrenic, made to clean the WCs with a razor blade until Lieutenant Laing put a stop to it. No, I am not making it up. The truth begins with two. And I cannot put the phone call down to an accident. I have never received another such phone call in thirty-two years.

Part of my work was to 'downgrade' out of the Army on psychiatric grounds soldiers that the Army did not want. They were downgraded automatically by virtue of being patients in the first place. But how much to downgrade on an eight-point scale? The degree of downgrading entailed issues of return to unit, retention in the Army in another unit, place or field of service, discharge from the Army, on what sort of pension (if any) and so forth. I never upgraded anyone as far as I can remember. Diagnosis and grading had an enormous impact on the life of any patient, all the way from discharge from the Army and direct transfer under certificate to a civilian mental hospital, with the prospect of lobotomy not far away, through to a 'free discharge' with some sort of financial back-up.

As far as I could make out, the strategy behind such grading of clinical status, with its economic and social implications, emanated from outside the medical branch of the British Army. I shall never know. Whom were we to 'discharge' back to their units or out of the service? One month we sent 10 per cent back and discharged 90 per cent; the next month we discharged 10 per cent and retained 90 per cent. It was up to the Army to determine how trimmed down they wanted to be. The Korean war was on. Manpower, conscription, morale presented problems.

Malingering could become a major issue, if one wanted to become too fastidious. A lot of soldiers seemed to be prepared to go to almost any lengths to get out.

How many soldiers were malingering their way out of the Army by kidding they were more or less daft? I got very interested in that problem. I do not know how many of those I saw as patients were up to this trick, or were a bit daft anyway and, with the benefit of a low IQ, were kidding they were dafter. They certainly were liable to get more than they had bargained they were letting themselves in for, especially if they were diagnosed as psychotic.

Three British officers captured by the Turks in World War I tell the story of how they got themselves repatriated by feigning madness to their Turkish captors. The Turks gave them a hard time. If anyone was trying it on all the way in the British Army, by the time the Army was through with them they deserved to get away with it.

One night when I was doing my late-night 'look in' on the ward, I happened to be caught by the ravings of a manic character coming from one of the padded cells.* I ordered an injection if he did not shut up soon.

I had the padded cell opened and went in and sat down to listen a bit more before he would have to be stopped by injection. He calmed down. I stayed for half an hour or so. He did not need an injection. On the next few nights I stayed for longer until I was almost 'hanging out' during the night with him in his padded cell. I felt strangely at home there, lounging on the floor.

This was the first time ever I really relaxed, settled down, in the company of any such patient without bothering to try to make sense of it, to diagnose the psychopathology in it, to interpret it or to try to infer from it, as a neurological symptom, what the underlying disorder to the central nervous system might be.

At first, I could *almost* understand him, I could *almost* follow. He was very fast.

He was in a padded cell because he had knocked himself out by taking a running jump, head first, at a brick wall. He could be anyone he cared to be merely by snapping his fingers. That was all right with me.

He could be anyone at all, but most of the time he was a gentleman catburglar and safe-blower in Manhattan or London or anywhere. He climbed through incredibly high, inaccessible windows, got into incredibly secure, locked rooms, got into vaults, blew up safes and made incredible getaways. The treasure, usually in gold and gems, was

---

* 'He' appears as John in my book *Self and Others*, Chapter 6.

distributed to the poor. He was never any the richer. I became his companion in some of these escapades. I was a sort of Sancho Panza to his Don Quixote.

After some weeks, when he had calmed down somewhat and was more reflexive, he nominated me Horatio to his Hamlet. He was soon discharged from the Army.

I had read Goldstein, Kasanin, Vigotsky *et al.* on schizophrenic thought-disorders. This was manic thought-disorder. But it did not seem quite to fit the textbooks: I had to listen for longer to make sure. These were the days before tape-recorders were in routine use, and I made no notes. If I had, I could not have followed what he was saying at the time. Anyway, this was not entirely a matter for clinical interest and research. It never occurred to me that it might be called therapy. It was beyond the line of duty. His padded cell had become a refuge for me and his company a solace.

It took me a few hours to catch up with his speed and when I was able to travel alongside him, as it were, my sensation that he was moving very fast evaporated. When I was moving at the same speed as him neither of us seemed to be moving particularly fast. He was flying around with his mind, like a bird – a very dangerous thing to do in such circumstances. He was already down for electric shocks like almost everyone, and, if his breakdown took on a schizophreniform complexion, insulin comas. The bird fluttered down to human form as Julius Caesar, Robin Hood, the Saint and others.

I have had occasion to see a number of people who were in padded cells.

What was going on here? What sort of thing was this? It was quite unlike *encephalitis lethargica* and the stuff neurologists see.

From notes at the time:

He is an Army officer of twenty-eight. He is cringing, naked, in the middle of a padded cell, wide awake day and night, twitching, quivering. He does not eat. He urinates and defecates where he crouches. He jabbers in fast *ratatatats* like bursts of machine-gun fire so that he is under continual machine-gun fire from all around, even, I seem to remember, the ground. He seems to us *completely* terrified. This utterly terrified creature pounces with reckless abandoned ferocity on anyone who tries to enter his padded cell.

He was going to die of exhaustion if he went on like that (no sleep, no food, no water): his terror did not seem to be doing him any good, so he had to be rushed away, sedated by intramuscular injection as often as necessary and to be tube-fed. He was transferred to a civilian hospital. I never heard what became of him.

He's a boxer. We're doing a ward round with the local chief psychiatrist, a lieutenant-colonel; I'm the intern. This Private So-and-So, he's suffering from aphonia: that is, he doesn't speak.

Three weeks ago he had a letter from his girlfriend saying that she was finished with him. He had stopped talking since receiving that letter. He had been struck dumb and paralysed by that information. He was now suffering from either catatonic or hysterical mutism – difficult to determine which.

Here's someone in a ward round who has stopped speaking for three weeks. He can't talk or he won't talk? Why is he dumb? Is he neurotic? Is he psychotic? Is he hearing voices? Is he malingering? Is he having us on? Is it organic or functional? Not only is he not talking but neither does he write.

'Finger up the arse, Sister; finger up the arse,' says the lieutenant-colonel. The ward-round procession moves on to the next patient.

He opened a letter from his fiancée. It was all off. He was

struck dumb. For over three weeks he was *speechless*. One
can get *cold feet*, literally. One can be *scared stiff*, literally.
One can get *a lump in one's throat*. I wonder why?

Peter was a private. A few months after being conscripted
into military service he broke down and ended up in the
ward in which I was working at Netley. He was a private
and I was a lieutenant.

He was of no use to the Army, so he would be given a
medical discharge. The only question was whether he
would first be transferred to the psychotic unit for insulin
and/or electric shocks, or to a civilian psychiatric unit for
the same sort of treatment.

I was just beginning to suspect that insulin and electric
shocks did more harm than good. In fact, I had begun to
have to call into question my own sanity, because I was
beginning to suspect that insulin and electric shocks, not to
mention lobotomy and the whole environment of a psychiatric unit, were ways of destroying people and driving
people crazy if they were not so before, and crazier if they
were. But I had to put it to myself – maybe I was completely
mistaken. How could the whole of psychiatry be doing the
opposite of what I assumed psychiatry was about – treating,
curing if possible, arresting the course of mental illness?
Was Artaud right?

Whichever way I turned, this issue became an almost
unbearable nightmare. Thirty-three years later it still is,
when I face the issues completely nakedly, as it were,
without taking some measure of comfort from anticipating
the conclusion to which I eventually came. Let me once
more try to start from scratch and put to you this conflict in
which I had become irremediably embroiled.

I was going on a week's leave to Glasgow. I knew that in
my absence Peter would almost certainly be transferred to
the insulin unit, or at least be given electric shocks. This
was the treatment that, from the clinical psychiatric point of
view, at that time and place at any rate, he required more

urgently as every day went by. Yet, between ourselves, he gave a much less schizophrenic impression in my office than he did on the ward. I could not bring myself to let that happen to him. How could I justify my arrogance with hardly any clinical psychiatric experience, in the face of the theory and practice of a massive part of modern medicine? Anyhow, rightly or wrongly, I decided to take him with me.

We travelled together and he slept in my bedroom at home. We were inseparable for three days until I went around to see a friend, Karl Abenheimer, one afternoon. I was away for three or four hours. When I got back he was curled up on his bed, in a corner. He stayed curled up there for the remaining four days of my week's leave and never said a word.

He swallowed tea and chocolates that my mother put in his mouth and went to the lavatory himself. When I had to go back to Netley, he got dressed and, still without a word but with impeccable behaviour, he accompanied me back.

I explained to him that all he had to do was to continue to walk, sit, stand and lie down in a normal way, to obey orders and speak (a few words would do) when spoken to, and he would be out of the Army for good in a few weeks. If he could not keep that much up, I could not guarantee that I could save him from electric shocks and maybe a diagnosis of schizophrenia and deep insulin before he could get out – and then, almost certainly, only to a civilian mental hospital.

We parted, he to the ward and me to the officers' mess, without him saying a word. He managed to keep up appearances and was duly 'invalided out' of the Army. When he did talk to me again after a week or so he said that when I left him he just went completely limp and helpless but somehow it was still all right. That was how it felt to me. I could see that from a psychiatric point of view he had lapsed into catatonic mutism, beset by God knows what obsessional paranoid ruminations and fantasies, and that any 'ordinary' psychiatrist would have had him 'admitted' right away. But the other side of me, the ordinary human being in me who found himself at the beginning of a psychiatric career, would have felt that to do so would have been to betray him completely. It was only in retrospect that I realized the full extent to which I did not accept psychiatric theory and practice and I began to realize that, with such an attitude, I was going to have a very strange professional career.

Years later, he became the director of a well-known college of dance and drama. He would have stood no chance whatsoever if he had gone through the usual psychiatric mill.

How can I justify such an opinion? What scientific evidence can I offer for such an outrageous statement?

I can offer no 'scientific' evidence. Neither is there any scientific evidence to suggest that psychiatric treatment would have done him more good than harm.

I developed an intense desire to be able to ferret out the differences between deception, malingering, self-deception (hysteria), neurosis and psychosis, functional and organic.

My first published paper was a study of a case that manifested this problem.*

A soldier was referred to the Royal Victoria Hospital, Netley, for a psychiatric opinion on his fitness to undergo trial by court-martial on a charge of desertion. He had been absent without leave for seven months. I had to make out a report. I interviewed the patient and other relevant people, consulted Army documents and constructed the following 'history'.

He was born after a normal pregnancy, his childhood and school years passed without any obviously unusual feature. He was never very bright. He had a younger brother and sister. His parents were both alive and in good health. Ten

* Published in the *Journal of the Royal Army Medical Corps*.

years earlier, after a few semi-skilled jobs, he had joined the regular Army as a private. He had a clean record.

He had married nine years earlier. He had a son. After several years during which he was abroad his wife had a child by another man and he divorced her. His wife kept their child.

A year before he came to Netley he had a road accident. He was not driving. He was in hospital for several months with severe chest injuries. No brain injuries were detected. In hospital he lay crying or saying nothing. When he got out of hospital, before returning to duty, his parents said he was a different man. He wandered in and out of their house. He was tearful and depressed. He went absent without leave a few weeks after returning to duty. He wandered around fair-grounds doing odd jobs. From time to time he arrived home, stayed a few days, borrowed some money. He seemed to them to be in a daze, 'not himself'. He hardly talked, complained of headaches and developed a marked stammer. He surrendered himself to the Army a few months later.

In prison, awaiting court-martial, he seemed peculiar. He was referred to a psychiatrist for a 'report on his mental condition'. On examination he was in tears for most of the interview, unable to speak because of a speech impediment, but said he wanted to kill himself. So he was admitted to Netley 'for observation'. That is where I came in. The following were my 'observations'.

On admission he said nothing. He was completely mute. He blew out his cheeks till he was blue in the face in prodigious efforts to utter even a whisper. He then cried, beat his head and tore his hair. He could write freely and indicated that he understood perfectly what I was saying to him.

An intravenous injection of pentothal seemed to be called for under the circumstances. The pentothal immediately released a torrent of obscene abuse against both his wife and the Army. He yelled himself hoarse in a few minutes, then burst out moaning and wailing and crying. 'Me Mom's good, me Mom's good, she's good she's good.' He enacted the driving accident, crying out, 'It's not my fault, not my fault.' After the session he again became mute, exactly as before.

In five subsequent sessions during the next three weeks he behaved in the same way. After the third session he talked with difficulty for a while and felt he was going blind. After the fifth session he talked fluently but felt weak, faint, dizzy, and had a splitting headache. The next day these symptoms disappeared, but he seemed to be in a confused state of anxious excitement. I put him on fairly heavy sedation; his anxiety became less evident. He had to be fed. He had to be taken to the toilet. He wanted to play with toys. He asked for a yo-yo.

Now he spoke without stuttering or stammering or puffing and blowing. But it was impossible to elicit a correct answer to the most simple questions. He said that two times two were two. He called an apple an orange. He said that leaves appeared on the trees in autumn, and gave the date, month and year incorrectly. He seemed to be speaking or whispering to his Mum a lot of the time. He seemed to see her, maybe to hear her. He said she was in the hospital. He said that he had been in hospital for months and that he was now in Chester. Mention of his wife, the Army, or almost anything might call out hilarious laughs, or he might growl, gnash his teeth, spit, and roar out obscene abuse. He was never actually violent.

He seemed to see his mother in the morning. He would whisper to her (with no speech impediment). He seemed to remove himself from the present and become a baby with his mother once more. He spent most of his time like this.

He did not respond to pin-pricks anywhere on his body (his whole body was analgesic). His hands had to be bandaged because of his practice of stubbing out cigarettes on them. He would fall into a deeply suggestible state at a mere word, but it was not possible to elicit a correct answer, even under hypnosis.

He gradually improved until, after six weeks, his parents did not find him recognizably different from his old self.

In 1897 Ganser, a German psychiatrist who specialized in this sort of situation – treating prisoners on remand – described what has become known as 'the Ganser Syndrome'. He characterized it as 'a specific hysterical twilight state, the chief symptom of which is *Vorbeireden* – talking past the point'. It is sometimes called the 'syndrome of approximate answers'. He noted this syndrome in prisoners on remand. All his cases were hallucinated. Many exhibited generalized analgesia. The condition always subsided within a few days.

The syndrome is regarded as a 'prison psychosis'. It is associated with hysterical 'pseudo-dementia' and hysterical puerilism. It was generally agreed that its main characteristic was the disappearance of the memory for elementary knowledge and experience, which remains intact in the organic disturbances.

Various suggestions have been put forward in an attempt to understand the meaning of this peculiar state. It occurs when the patient, 'although mentally deranged, not realizing this, wishes to appear so'. Some think that many Ganser states may be schizoid reaction psychoses. The patient, being under charges from which he would be exonerated were he irresponsible, begins, without being aware of the fact, to appear irresponsible. It has been suggested that this 'psycho-physiological regression to the unconscious level' is 'available to all patients entering upon mental illness, and utilized as a drastic attempt at self-reorganization'.

I was fascinated that, in the course of observation and investigation-treatment (mental examinations, the so-called truth drug pentothal narcosis, hypnosis), my soldier-patient had developed a full-blown 'syndrome' that fitted exactly, in both symptoms and circumstances, the 'syndrome' described by Ganser. The 'precipitating factor' was the removal of the hysterical speech inhibition. The patient tried to restrict the range of the thinkable to one subject alone – the Good Mother ('I shall think of me Mom alone for a thousand years and nothing else'). He regressed to the age of two or three, he incorporated orally his Good Mother and projected his psychic reality to the external world ('Me Mom's here'). All studies of the condition agree that the 'paralogia' is not entirely consciously determined.

The paralogia, the regression, the confused, disorientated consciousness, the wholesale denial of unpleasant external reality, the hallucinosis, the generalized analgesia, together seem to constitute a peculiar constellation of defences that are not constitutionally available to everyone. Was the patient 'fit to plead'?

During my time at Netley I began to think for the first time, seriously, that there might be (as Harry Stack Sullivan argued) a *mésalliance* between neurology and psychiatry – at least that aspect of psychiatry that was beginning to capture most of my attention. I realized that if this were so I was going to be in for a terrible time of it, because I was already beginning to feel that it was imperative for me either to clarify this confusion or to discover that there was not after all the confusion I suspected. This was a prospect from which I cringed, because I already knew the terrible pain of conflicting, clashing intellectual allegiances within my own mind. At the same time, I counted myself very fortunate that my mind had found a problem upon which it had full scope to exhaust itself. I also had to accept the possibility that I might think and work myself into a hopeless mess. And always, in the meantime, all this mass of unalleviated human misery, a large part of which, I was beginning to suspect, was being manufactured by psychiatry itself.

I still felt, however, that there was the possibility of a proper alliance between the study of disordered brains and disordered minds and interpersonal relations: through such an alliance, neuroscience could contribute to lessening personal and interpersonal forms of human misery.

Personal and interpersonal misery cuts across the divisions between biology, neurology and psychiatry. Take head injuries. Someone sustains a severe head injury. He is knocked unconscious and stays unconscious, in coma, for days, weeks, months. He is kept alive by a life-support system provided by a neurosurgical unit. He eventually comes round. It is a well-known clinical observation that the character who 'comes round' may bear *no* more resemblance to the chap who was there before the head injury than to Tom, Dick or Harry. The post-traumatic personality may not even remember the pre-traumatic personality. Over a period of months the post-traumatic personality learns who he is, and who everyone and what everything is, by being told. Some functions come back effortlessly, others never.

There are intimate links between the state of our central nervous systems and our minds, our very selves.

Such an injury to the head might not cause even a fracture of a bone. It might not even cause any bleeding. It stuns the brain, which functions very little, hardly at all, almost not at all. Coma. Eventually we may start to come round. We may not recognize anyone. We may have no idea who we are, or were. Others, whom we do not know, tell us. It is clear that neurological changes can evoke such changes in personality and communication. It is therefore perfectly reasonable to speculate about and to try to determine what neurological disturbances there may be when we come across disturbed interpersonal communication.

After a year at Netley, I was transferred to Northern Command at Catterick in Yorkshire. I became a captain and had the job of being, in effect, in clinical and administrative command of the psychiatric ward and the detention ward of Catterick Military Hospital, which contained any sort of prisoners in detention in any sort of medical or surgical condition, psychiatric or not. The two wards were separated by steel grilles, the detention ward being doubly secured behind a double-locked grille and two double-locked doors. These wards were my domain. In addition, my duties included any sort of psychiatric referral. I liaised with the rest of the hospital in terms of neurological, neuropsychiatric problems, had to visit various units in Northern Command, to visit and give a psychiatric report on any soldier on whom it was deemed appropriate who had got into a civilian prison . . .

The ear-nose-and-throat specialist at Catterick was Murray Brookes, now Professor of Clinical Research at Guy's Hospital, London. He was sure that many of the soldiers whose ears and auditory functions he was examining could hear perfectly well. Were they malingering? He sent a few to me. It is a difficult clinical problem. A soldier suddenly does not hear the sergeant-major, or anyone else. If he keeps it up, even half convincingly, he will have to be referred to the medical officer, who will have to refer him to the ear-nose-and-throat specialist, who will have to refer him to a psychiatrist. The two of us would have to come to a decision. We wrote a paper on this subtle clinical problem, which was turned down by the editors of the *Journal* of the RAMC.

Someone may claim that he is *partially*, or 'only sometimes', deaf in one ear, maybe both, he's not sure, it comes and goes; sometimes it's as though both ears are plugged with cotton wool. Sometimes everything sounds far away, sometimes there is a ringing noise. And fainting? What is a 'genuine' faint on a parade ground? How can one tell whether someone has a splitting headache or not? The diagnosis could vacillate from malingering to hysteria to a brain tumour or brain abscesses or encephalitis.

The ear-nose-and-throat specialist and I did a study of simulated, functional, hysterical and organic deafness. He had some tricks to catch out people who were trying to catch him out, but, with or without such tricks and traps, I had to conclude that I could not tell whether someone was lying, or telling the truth, or somewhere in between. I did not know anyone who could, or how one could.

The complaint of deafness is fairly frequent and interesting because deceit can often be proved objectively. Deafness as the presenting symptom of a psychotic illness is uncommon. As an hysterical conversion symptom it is a comparative rarity.

Soldiers complain of all types and degrees of deafness. There may be a discoverable organic basis. If not, someone is reporting a sensation to which no correlative physical signs can be found. The condition is 'functional', the patient is 'neurotic' or lying. If he is not lying he is in some way ill, but his illness is not a pathological process in his body. He needs help.

A dysfunction of the auditory sphere could be the expression of an upset of the total personality. Disturbances of hearing occur in hysteria, in anxiety states, in inhibitory reactions to catastrophic psychic traumata, in schizophrenia, etc. The psychiatrist sorts these various forms of functional deafness into categories. Deafness can also be simulated. The patient is lying. How can one tell? A malingerer, who is lying, makes statements he himself believes to be false. He simulates something to be the matter. He is not deceiving himself. He does not himself believe that he suffers from his disability. He has to be on his guard constantly. It is not easy to lie consistently for long.

The presence or absence of anxiety does not help us to differentiate forms of functional deafness, nor to distinguish functional deafness, as a class, from malingering.

I am not concerned here with the character-structure of the malingerer – why some people take this course to evade military service or an unpleasant situation, and others do not. Is the diagnosis mendacity or veracity? The extreme difficulty of deciding is illustrated by the following case.

A man of twenty was brought to hospital 'in hysterics' –
screaming, shouting, throwing himself about. He had just
wrecked the barrack room where he lived. He rapidly
quietened down in hospital. He said he had had a pain
in his ears so intense that it drove him to smash things up to
escape it. He had had a similar experience fourteen months
before entering the Army, and once before that in childhood. He had no parents. We could not confirm or dis-
confirm his story. A thorough examination of his central
nervous system, including radiography and electro-en-
cephalography, and ontological and psychiatric investigation revealed no abnormalities. Only once during his spell
in hospital did he have a recurrence of pain in his ears,
when it had been mentioned that he would soon be discharged to his unit. Was this man lying or not?

A disease may be simulated in four ways. One can falsify
the past; falsify what one feels; artificially produce signs
suggesting a disease from which one does not suffer; kid
oneself daft. There are 'fits' no one has seen and which no
one can remember because of black-outs. All sorts of
complaints: 'I can't think clearly. I feel different.'

Another patient was noticeably agitated and nervous. He
had been deaf, he said, since childhood, but never had
scarlet fever or mumps. He did not seem to have complained about being deaf however until he had been a few
weeks in the Army. It did not interfere with school or with
earning a living on leaving school. No one else in the family
was deaf. He said his ears had been running for years,
though they looked normal through an otoscope.

Some people are suddenly totally stone deaf in one ear.

When challenged, bilateral deafness could become uni-
lateral, Rinne-negative become Rinne-positive. The Weber
test might correctly lateralize, the Schwabach test demonstrate the integrity of the inner ear, and stone deafness
would become mild.

A regular recruit, two weeks in the Army, said he had had
difficulty in hearing 'for a considerable time'. His father

wore a hearing aid and was receiving a pension for deafness. His brother was receiving a pension for deafness.

Nothing showed up on tests. He had difficulty in hearing words in either ear in a loud voice at ten feet. He could only hear half the words. He gave clang associations to them. He heard 'death' as 'collapse'. He never had the slightest difficulty in hearing me in ordinary conversation. He was discharged from the Army, quickly.

We kept 'in' another man who had been deaf in one ear for six weeks. Now he could not hear the sergeant on parade. 'When they fire .303s, everything goes blurred.' After three weeks in the Army, his deafness was very bad. He was examined. We told him he was not deaf. He burst into tears: 'My mother is in hospital for three weeks; my poor father has to do all the work on his own. If only I could help him, even in the evenings.' He had four younger sisters.

We would have been better to let him go, I suppose.

One always had to be on the alert. One could never tell. Just before I was due to go off on weekend leave to Glasgow, I was asked to look at a chap from a medical ward who was pushed in front of me in a wheelchair screaming his head off, panting between screams that he had an excruciating headache. The physician in charge of the medical ward, a fellow conscript and captain of my age, had examined him neurologically and could detect nothing unequivocally abnormal. Was he under intracranial pressure (which he almost had to be if his screams were to be believed), or was he 'hysterical' or something like that, or was he malingering or what? I had a quick look at him. I tried to look at his pupils, but he kept his eyes tightly shut. His temperature was normal. He did not seem ill, apart from his screaming. His tendon reflexes were not grossly exaggerated or absent or asymetrical.

He would not, or could not, get out of his chair . . . ? I was pretty fed up by now with malingerers. He might well be another of them – more than likely. I was on the verge of ordering him to stand up or be stood up, but I gave him the benefit of the doubt. I ordered him to be wheeled back to the ward and recommended he be kept under close clinical observation. I told my medical colleague that I did not know what was wrong and – caught my train.

When I got back on Monday morning he was dead. The medical specialist decided to give him a lumbar puncture when he got back to the ward and drew out thick pus. He had meningeal encephalitis with a vengeance. They poured in penicillin but it was too late and he was dead in a few hours.

The issue of malingering colours not only the Army's but everyone's attitude to a psychiatric patient.

I collected a series of over sixty so-called 'attempted suicides' or 'suicidal gestures' before or after admission – by swallowing razor blades, nuts and bolts, soap, broken glass, lavatory chains, buttons, knives, forks, spoons, hair, hammers, files, combs, broken saws, coins, lavatory paper, clothing. At one juncture the commanding officer of the hospital ordered that absolutely every such object, except really tough pyjamas and trousers, be banished from the psychiatric ward, including buttons, and also soap and toilet rolls, which could only be handed out specifically on request at the discretion of the staff. For several weeks previously anything that appeared on the ward had been eaten up. The surgeons had some practice in excavating such objects from stomachs and guts.

After about a week both the commanding officer and the patients seemed to relent and call it a day. He relaxed his orders, de-escalation was successful. The epidemic of 'attempted suicides' evaporated.

But were they all malingering? When can a person be regarded as psychotic?

Example: the Iron Man
He was a conscript in the British Army, aged eighteen, admitted to the psychiatric ward of Catterick Military

Hospital. It had been ascertained and confirmed by X-ray that he had an incredible bulk and variety of *iron* in his alimentary tract – a whole junk yard. He claimed he needed a lot of iron inside him to give him the strength necessary for Army life. He was going to be a man of iron. Was he just making up a story to 'kid he was daft'? If so he was a malingerer, but he would have to be psychopathic in some way to malinger like that. Not depressed. Not suicidal. Not manic. Not schizophrenic. Not obsessive. He did not swallow the iron compulsively. He talked about it in a calm, ordinary, matter-of-fact way, until he stopped talking and moving, becoming speechless and motionless. Malingering or mute catatonic immobility? Very curious.

The neck of the woods in which I had ended up for a mere two years was a place of misery, absurdity and humiliation. In my room in the officers' quarters, in the middle of the night, I would picture those other places, those barracks, those prisons, those other lunatic wards, those extermination wards, all those places of groans and tears that each night covers.

FIVE

The Mental Hospital

When I came out of the British Army in 1953, aged twenty-six, I had learned what was expected of a psychiatrist in the Army. It was much more than the exercise of a straightforward clinical, medical judgement, and in the treatment of patients something very different from ordinary, straightforward medicine or surgery. The decisions I had been called upon to make, and the commands to which I had had to respond, entailed all sorts of man-management, administration, organizational institutional power and structure, that had nothing to do with clinical medicine. I could see very clearly, I thought, the 'contingent necessity' for all that, but I had not read about it in the psychiatric textbooks and I could only bluff my way along when, by virtue of being a psychiatrist, I was consulted by a commanding officer about morale under his command. I knew I had no competence to advise about that sort of thing, but he assumed I had. During World War II, psychiatrists in the Army had come to be specialists in the maintenance in good order of the human 'software': human relations – in other words, on advising the Army on the economic use of manpower. Avoid square pegs in round holes. What good was all the hardware in the world, unless the software, the human material, could be used effectively? How does this type of psychiatric thinking affect clinical practice?

What sort of creature is a psychiatrist supposed to be? I was now drawn deeply into the complexities and confusions of psychiatry, and went from the Army to work in Glasgow's Gartnavel Royal Mental Hospital.

Army psychiatry was not concerned with long-term custodial care. In Gartnavel there were patients who had been 'in' for ten, thirty, sixty years: since the nineteenth century.

I was allocated to the female side of the hospital. After two years of men in the Army, I was glad to be among women.

A refractory ward in a mental hospital is a strange place to be reminded of Homer. But these women in the refractory ward brought back to me Homer's description of the ghosts in Hades, separated on their side from the living by the width of the Ocean, and, on the part of the living, by the Rivers of Fear. Ulysses goes to the land of the dead to meet his mother. Although he can see her, he is dismayed to find he cannot embrace her. She explains to him that she has no sinews, no bones, no body keeping the bones and flesh together. Once the life force has gone from her white bones, all is consumed by the fierce heat of a blazing fear, and the soul slips away like a dream and flutters in the air.

From what experience of life had that description come? It seemed to be so far and yet so near.

How can we entice these ghosts to life, across *their* oceanic abyss, across *our* rivers of fear?

In the refractory ward was an old lady who had been hospitalized with episodic manic attitudes at regular intervals for over twenty years. She was a spinster who, when not manic, devoted her life to church mission work: in the slums with unmarried mothers, prostitutes and girls who would probably become prostitutes. In the refractory ward she was one of them, all of them. In between, she ranted and roared and raved. She was massively indignant at the doctors who had raped her, impregnated her, forced her to have hundreds of babies or abortions and given her syphilis. If not raging about the vicious sexual horrors that had been visited upon her, she might be miserable or merry. She never ceased in the least to pace about. Sometimes she would *prance* up and down.

After a while she overcame her fear of me and would sit and talk with me about all that sort of thing indefinitely, inexhaustibly. Once, when she was most distraught, I asked her, 'Why are you like this?' She suddenly stopped all her 'nonsense', and said in an intense but quite ordinary voice and with a face crucified by, racked by wretchedness and despair: 'Read Psalm 32, verses 3 and 4. I stuck at the Resurrection.' She then resumed her customary manner.

These are the verses she told me to read:

When I kept silence, my bones waxed old through my roaring all the day long.

For day and night thy hand was heavy upon me: my moisture is turned into the drought of summer.

I told her I had looked it up – sorry, that I had had to – and repeated it to her. She was touched. Her manic agony took on a different quality. It became more of an act. She continued for several weeks to keep it up with others, assiduously, and then only when a 'senior' member of staff entered the ward – assistant-matron level and up, on the nursing side, or, on the male side, any psychiatrist. Most of the time she would sit down beside me and we would silently survey the scene we were in together. From time to time, spontaneously, or when I asked her to, she would elucidate for me what this patient was doing, standing, immobile, all day, staring at the sky, and what that one was doing. She took me on. She became my mentor.

The female refractory ward was the ward, with padded cells, reserved for the very 'worst' patients. I sat in the day-room of this ward for one or two hours each day for several months. There were more than fifty patients up and about in the day-room. Most of them sat huddled in chairs, talking to no one, not even themselves, being spoken to by no one. However, these were not the patients one noticed first.

I think the first thing that happened to me when I had sat myself in a chair was that several patients fought each other to hug me or kiss me, to sit on my lap, to put their arms around me. They ruffled my hair, pulled my tie. I got my trouser buttons ripped open. I had to fight for my life sometimes with the two or three nurses on the spot in the ward to help me.

The patients queued in the mornings to have their hospital nightdresses whipped off and hospital day-gowns put on. Most of them had been in hospital for years. Most of them had had electric shocks and insulin to no avail. Several had had lobotomies. This was the end of the line.

My psychiatric presuppositions had prepared me for the autism of the patients. For the most part, they all seemed to be living in their own worlds. This was true in a sense but as time went on I realized it was only one side of the coin. There were a few patients with whom one did not need to speak in schizophrenese. My remitted manic patient sat by me often and explained to me a great deal of what went on. She told me that that patient, for instance, huddled in the far corner of the ward, gazing fixedly out a window, was furious that I had not looked at her when I had entered the ward. That patient curled up under a table, she told me, had been playing at being a snake for years.

At first the ward sounded like an out-of-tune orchestra endlessly tuning up, each instrument unrelated and out of pitch. With some acclimatization, it began to dawn on me that the autism of each patient, although autistic, was interwoven with that of the others. A more appropriate analogy seemed with the illumination that comes when the jumble of sound in a difficult piece of music all suddenly makes sense.

It did not make total sense, but I had glimpses when I felt it might. They were not exclusively self-absorbed. Some of them were literally paralysed, I realized, by being so absorbed in what was going on in their vicinity. The ward was terribly overcrowded. The nurses were harassed and overworked. The patients had nothing to do. The milieu was not 'therapeutic', although 'spontaneous' remissions did occur. I wanted to see what would happen if we could have a few patients together with the same nurses day after day for long enough, in less distressing surroundings but with everything else being equal.

Dr Angus MacNiven, the superintendent, and the matron gave me permission to try out an experiment in the management of a few of these chronic patients. Eleven patients and two nurses would be given a room to themselves from nine to five, Mondays to Fridays. The nurses would be assigned to these patients rather than to a ward. This idea was put into effect and kept going for a year after I left.

Eleven patients were selected from the most apparently withdrawn people in the ward. All were schizophrenics who had been in the same ward for over four years: their ages ranged from twenty-two to sixty-three. Matron delegated two nurses whose sole job was to be with these eleven patients. A large, bright, newly-decorated, comfortably furnished room was made available, in which were magazines, material for knitting and sewing, rug- and blanket-making, drawing and other pastimes. I gave no direct instructions to the nurses except to ask for daily written reports (which I allowed to lapse after a few weeks) and sociograms to be completed. I met the two nurses at least once a week to talk with them about the patients and I also paid informal visits to the room when they were there with the patients. The patients were in the room from nine a.m. to twelve noon and two to five p.m. except on Saturdays and Sundays.

On the first day, the eleven 'completely withdrawn' patients had to be shepherded from the ward across to the day-room. The second day, at half past eight in the morning, I had one of the most moving experiences of my life on that ward. There they all were clustered around the locked door, just waiting to get out and get over there with the two nurses and me. And they hopped and skipped and twiddled around and whatnot on their way over. So much for being 'completely withdrawn'.[8]

The patients were much 'better behaved' than they were in the ward. There was no sense of threat of real physical danger. The nurses were not too harassed. The room had not that smell of hopeless terror that was in the refractory ward.

In that room, it became ever more clear to me that these patients were exquisitely sensitive to nuances that some people never notice, or dismiss as petty. They are always there and far from petty. Most of us walk over them but some people drown in them, patients or not.

A doctor visits the ward. He smiles at the charge nurse, speaks to her in a whisper, signs the report book and then strolls round the ward with her. This is his daily, literal ward round. A patient makes a dash at the doctor. She is barred by the female charge nurse. She accuses the nurse bitterly of standing between her and the doctor, as she is doing. Some patients are frightened that the doctors will take their nurses away from them.

After being 'around' in the ward or the room for a while, my entrance or exit ceased to be an event. A nurse told me that to begin with they had mixed feelings about my visits because the patients had previously been noisy and excited during and after my visits, but now they were not so. She put this down to the fact that now they had become so used to me that they did not have to interrupt what they had been doing – say, standing still and concentrating (exhibiting the signs of catatonic mutism).

Perhaps the most difficult time came when the nurses started to get fond of the patients as people, instead of sorry for them as patients. They worried that the other nurses

might think they were having a cushy job. They worried
that they were actually enjoying themselves sometimes,
with the patients. There must be some mistake.

After several months, after a lot of heart-searching,
matron and superintendent overruled misgivings and allowed the nurses and patients to have a gas stove and oven.
They could now make tea for themselves. This was un-
thinkable in the ward (danger of pouring scalding water
over themselves or drinking it, etc.). They made tea and
they made some buns. Ian Cameron, one of the psychiatrists, took some of the buns over to the doctors' sitting
room and offered them round. There were seven or eight of
us psychiatrists sitting around. Only two or three were
brave, or reckless, enough to eat a bun baked by a chronic
schizophrenic.

This incident convinced me of something. Who was
crazier? Staff or patients? Excommunication runs deep.
A companion means, literally, one with whom one shares
bread. Companionship between staff and patients had
broken down. The psychiatrists were afraid of catching
schizophrenia. Who knows? It might be contagious, like
herpes, through mucous membranes.

In the room, the patients were now all wearing under-
wear, dresses, stockings and shoes. They coiffured their
hair and some wore make-up. They were recognizably
ordinary human beings again, however daft they were.
One lady was exhausted at the end of every day, having
to look after five children invisible and inaudible to all but
her.

Within eighteen months all original eleven patients had
left hospital. Within a further year, they were all back. Had
they found more companionship 'inside' than they could
find 'outside'?

I still did not want neurology and psychiatry to fall apart for
me. I had never lost touch with neurology through the
friendship that developed between Joe Schorstein and me,

and I now wanted to focus on something 'clinical' which could keep it all together. We ran a headache clinic together for a year.

The interpersonal processes in the recovery from head injury seemed a strategic point on which to focus. I so much wanted my interpersonal and neurological interests to be married, not to be divorced from each other.

After severe brain damage, an individual may be reduced to a state of helplessness, which requires a life-support system sustained for a prolonged period by unremitting nursing care. For weeks, even months, all thoughts, memory, imagination, intentions, feelings and actions may be, or may seem to be, virtually wiped out as a result of physical brain damage. During recovery, sometimes over a period of years, these functions re-emerge: patterns re-form and recrystallize.

After severe concussion, coma, amnesia, the person who re-emerges may hardly bear any resemblance to what he or she was like before. A post-traumatic personality appears which is often quite unlike the pre-traumatic personality, before the brain was damaged. This is a difficult neurological problem. How do we account for it in neurological terms? How do these changes within the person, and his or her reassimilation of and reabsorption into the world of others correlate with neurological events? I wanted to see how interpersonal and neurological recovery intermeshed to generate the emergence of a new personality.

A brain injury knocks out all interpersonal processes along with the rest, and recovery entails some degree of interpersonal style. However, interpersonal style is far too vague a concept to be of much use neurologically. Neurologically one can study memory and other mental functions in various organic conditions. 'Personality' is another kettle of fish.

There was something very puzzling about this problem. For I became aware that if I looked at someone neurologically, his or her personality tended to fade from view, into the background, and, conversely, if I regarded someone personally who was not obviously physically impaired, the neurological point of view tended to disappear. For instance, I would see someone smile, not various facial muscles contracting and relaxing.

Interpersonal relationships are not found on neurological examination. We do not see consciousness down a microscope. We see brain cells. People with great handicaps, blindness, deafness, aphasias, paralysis may get on very well with their fellows. Many severe organic lesions do not seem to impair the capacity to relate as person to person – a very convenient complex set of skills to have at one's disposal. How may the ability to form and experience a human bond with human beings be impaired neurologically? How do the ways our brains function affect the ways we love, hate and generally relate to each other?

As movements and actions come back after coma and paralysis, at some stage, sometimes quite suddenly, with a few scattered movements, a body strikes everyone around as a fellow human being again.

But when does a body become a person? How can we answer that question? Is it a subtle perceptual illusion? When and how did a 'he', a 'she', a 'you' re-emerge? This re-emergence seems to coincide with the moment that *we* feel *addressed* by a him, a her, a you, not merely reacted *to* by an *it*. I wanted to approach this moment in terms of some vision of a possible interpersonal neurology of it.

We construe another person's relation to ourselves, to him- or herself, from his or her speech and conduct. Brain damage may wipe out, for a while, all speech and conduct. Until expressive sound and movements return we are without access to what such a brain-damaged person's relations to his or her self may be, if any. There is a qualitative discontinuity between the sense of no one there and the *recognition* of someone there; there is a very convincing moment of recognition of another person again. We feel another presence again.

This *presence*, so immediate to our sensibility, of the other eludes being pinned down entirely objectively. A few moments ago there was just a body making a few movements. Now, someone is *there*. The moment we snap into this sense of the immediate presence of the other, movements express intentions, and we are back in the realm of human *conduct*, however vestigial. Our sense of the presence of the other endows his or her movements with meaning. We may be wrong.

This moment of recognition of the other may coincide with the first time *we* feel 'looked at' by the other 'coming around'. We feel the other feels us.

The moment is the great divide between *before*, when there is little more than a heart-lung preparation lying there, and *after*, when someone is there again.

When the post-traumatic personality is compared to the pre-traumatic personality, 'it' is often characterized, clinically, as somewhat 'disinhibited', less aware of the nuances of other people's sensibilities: excessively euphoric, aggressive, rude, etc. The brain damage is taken to have knocked out this or that 'inhibiting' centre. There is an old neurosurgical dictum that after a head injury one is inclined to become more of a child and less of an adult.

This neurological 'regression' after head injury is different from what is called 'regression' in psychiatry – and yet biological and psychological regression do seem to have something more than a name in common.

Nan was fifteen when she ran out of school one lunch-break into the path of a grey car which tossed her high in the air. She landed in the path of a second car, travelling in the opposite direction, which came to a stop over her. She sustained severe head injuries, and lay in a coma like a vegetable for two months.

Before her accident she was described as a dutiful, conscientious, hardworking, somewhat fussy schoolgirl, who devoted herself to helping her mother manage the house and to looking after four younger brothers and sisters.

After eight months in hospital she emerged as a playful, lighthearted, likeable coquette, though fragile, easily upset and frightened.

After another six months at home, she changed further. She became sad, a little embittered that her school friends had left her behind. She could not go out alone and have a good time like the other girls. She was readily irritated and would lose her temper if she did not get her own way. She could dress herself, walk unassisted. She helped her mother a little by dusting and washing dishes. She was impish and flirtatious in ways others found inoffensive and rather endearing.

Nan had lain curled up like an almost dead, unborn baby for six weeks after her accident. She had to be tube-fed until she could be spoonfed and then, after three months, she began to be able to co-ordinate her hand-to-mouth movements enough to feed herself.

She was motionless and expressionless for six weeks. No personality was in evidence. How did a 'personality' come to be in evidence again? Nan was limp (atonic) and mute. No movements, no words, no recognition, no 'personal' reactions.

Her first movements were very limited. She could open and shut her eyes, contract her forehead, open and shut her mouth, bring her right hand to her mouth, move her trunk and legs a little.

These movements were taken by some of those about her to be *expressions*, whereas they appeared to others to be no more than involuntary contractions of various muscles or muscle groups. A contraction of the forehead looks like a frown. A wave of contractions of the muscles of her face gives the impression she is tired, or irritable. Even the most seasoned clinician has an involuntary tendency to react to such presumably involuntary movements as though they are 'voluntary'. This takes us into the problems of the

Gestalt perception of human beings. When does a still or changing or moving form look like a human face? Could it be that some people do not actually perceive people, but things?

These first movements were seized upon by those closest as evidence that 'she' was coming round and back. Eyelids droop. Is there a 'she' behind them who is tired? What sort of existence has such a 'she', or any 'he', 'you' or 'me'? A mouth opens. Is there a 'she' who is hungry?

One hundred and forty-two days after her accident, I was sitting by her bed. With some help, leaning to her left, she rested her head on the bed-rail, rubbing her forehead against it. She slowly brought her right hand across and gripped the rail with it. She stayed like that for two minutes then let herself fall back, and as she lay she seemed quite exhausted by her effort. She opened her mouth wide several times. After a few minutes some energy seemed to come back. She started to agitate the blankets with her legs, shook them off, succeeded in putting both her legs over the rail and began to swing her feet backwards and forwards as they hung from her knees on the rail. She stroked my knee as the pendulum swung. I withdrew my knee slightly. She augmented the swing of her legs to keep the touch of the very light stroke. After several swings she just managed to withdraw her legs into the bed before she was once more completely exhausted for another few minutes. In her next effort she contrived to put both her legs (so emaciated were they) between the same two rails. When I pressed the soles of her feet to induce her to withdraw her legs she said 'No' but then allowed her legs to be put back. As I rested my arm on the bed-rail while she lay on her back, she lifted herself up and stroked it with her forehead.

Thus, from the very first, her movements were framed by us doctors around her, both neurologically and personally. The nurses, her visitors, lacking any training in adopting the neurological point of view, just saw 'her'. Their perception of her movements as human 'reads' an intention into them, and seems to draw a personality out of them. Is this our invention? That mouth opens again. Does 'she' want sweets? This is not apparent to me, nor to the neurologists. The nurses use 'her' craving for sweets to have 'her' *take* sweets from them. It is not a matter of popping sweets into a buccal cavity. They are 'giving' 'her' sweets; '*she*' was 'taking' sweets. They pet 'her'. They do not rub a piece of skin. They try to get 'Nan' to do this and that. They coax 'her' and stroke 'her' hair.

Her first 'smiles' were slow, 'viscid', waxing and waning movements. Suddenly there was a strong impression that 'she' was trying to smile. 'She' seemed 'to smile' when 'she' seemed at a loss. Her 'smile' was warmly encouraged. People would try to coax her to smile by putting out their tongues, making funny faces.

The new 'Nan' at first was the 'Nan' that other people made out of the opening and shutting of her eyes, the contracting of her forehead, the opening and shutting of her mouth and so on.

When her speech began to come back, people tended to make allowances for her impairments by treating her speech defects as jokes and wit. Again a human intention was ascribed before, to the neurological ear or eye, any intention was apparent and, very likely, before any intention was *there*.

Her first utterances seemed quite incongruous and off the mark. It was a considerable time before it was convincing that she had a fairly adequate understanding of what was said and meant what she said herself. In the meantime people decided that she was a bit of a wit and a few jumbled words were a joke. When 'she' had come back, to everyone's ordinary perception and satisfaction, 'she' quickly took up this cue and played up to the part of being 'a proper card' for all she was worth.

The girl whom almost everyone had given up for dead had come back to life. She was unashamedly 'spoiled'. Her hair was always carefully arranged, decorated by a ribbon.

The nurses loved to powder her face and put on lipstick. She was always being told how pretty and clever she was. Whether 'she' seemed vain, coy, impish, coquettish, forward or cheeky, all was welcome, indulged, encouraged. All this sort of thing that was going on between her and the nurses seemed to be very important in her recovery indeed – vital to, essential to the very stuff and essence of her recovery – and yet it all went outside the usual field of vision of neuroscience. It cannot be described in neurological terms alone, nor in terms of a combination of neurology and some variety of behavioural conditioning theory, because what had to be seen to be described was not the reappearance of reflexes or the emergence of a new set of conditioned responses, but a new person. We cannot see a person if we see in a human being *only* sets of conditioned reflexes and responses. Could this perception of a 'person' be another illusion, at any time?

The new 'Nan' began as a construction by the others. 'She' was the significance of, the meaning of, 'she' was what they made of the openings and shuttings of her eyes, contractions of facial muscles, openings and shuttings of her mouth, unco-ordinated jerks of her hand. These contractions and jerks were read as attempts at gestures and expressions when 'neurologically' they were still read as 'involuntary'. The *assimilation* of these neurologically non-personal movements into a personal form seemed crucial in the formation of a new personality. They were endowed with meaning before they had a meaning in themselves. There was so little to go on that everyone was especially quick to see in any sign of life from that face, those fingers, an individual unity, to address as 'Nan'.

As her verbal ability developed Nan accepted and tried to fill out the rôle of playing to the gallery and *saw herself* as a bit of a wit, which she had never been before.

Such reactions to the ways others treated her rapidly congealed, as it were, to become fixed, indeed rigid, autonomous, established traits of a post-traumatic personality.

She seemed to build herself up on them and to elaborate them into a post-traumatic rôle as rather vain, impish, coquettish, rather useless but likeable. She learned to build upon this foundation other complementary patterns of behaviour that, as it were, 'fitted in' with the original basis. In this way her rôle was developed autonomously and she began to gain control over the reactions of others. If at first she was almost passively induced into a rôle provided and defined by others, she quickly became adept at *using* the 'new' personality they gave her to manipulate them. Her relationships with others became more *dialectic*. This process continued until she had a sufficiently stable and adequate set of patterns through which to interact with others and through which she could maintain a personal and social equilibrium between her impaired functions and the demands and expectations of others. Thus was formed her post-traumatic personality.

SIX

The Department of Psychiatry

I left Gartnavel Royal Mental Hospital in 1955 to take a National Health Service job as senior registrar at the Southern General Hospital, where the Department of Psychoogical Medicine of Glasgow University was located. I was the youngest, I was told, to hold that rank in Britain at the time. I was very keen and eager and getting into deeper and deeper waters. I was beginning to write my first book, *The Divided Self.* I was still trying to clarify what puzzled and upset me about neurology, neuropsychiatry, psychiatry. I was made a link-man between the psychiatric department and the other medical departments.

The Department of Psychiatry was approached by a group of ministers who wanted to be given a course on human relations, interpersonal theory, counselling and so on. The professor took the group – seven Protestant ministers of different denominations and a Rabbi – once a week, with me as his assistant. This experience drove home to me how little my psychiatric experience, limited as it was to the wards of either a mental hospital or a psychiatric unit in a general hospital and to out-patient clinics, could offer me in terms of knowing what was going on out there in the real world from which my patients came and to which they returned and in which they lived. These ministers not only had far more experience of actual human relations than I had, but they had more than I was ever going to acquire if I spent all my working days and nights in wards or consulting rooms, behind a desk, in my white coat with stethoscope, tendon hammer, pocket torch and ophthalmoscope.

I had to give them an account of Freud's theories on

separation, loss, grief, mourning, and melancholia. It had never occurred to me that some sort of grief and mourning was not the usual response to bereavement. If it did not appear, then I automatically interpreted that as a manic defence. All the ministers, however, quickly agreed between themselves from their extensive experience of death, funerals and the reactions of the deceased's nearest and dearest that, although some people were sad, unhappy, inclined to be given to depression and feelings of guilt when someone close died, they were not sure that they should regard such grief and mourning as the rule. Many people were made very relieved and much happier by a death. Handkerchiefs might be used to cover lack of emotion, or to conceal an embarrassing absence of sobs.

One minister told, for instance, of how in Aberdeen, walking with the husband of a Darby-and-Joan couple away from the grave in which his wife had just been buried, the husband turned to him and remarked, 'You know, I've lived with that woman fifty years, and I never liked her.' This anecdote evoked a ripple of understanding around his fellow ministers.

The answers to why a lot of people are in hospital are to be found only outside hospital. I had gone to medical school to learn about 'life'. I had dissected corpses, attended the ill and dying and the disturbed in mind. I realized how little I knew of real life.

What do you do when you don't know what to do? No wonder there are more suicides among psychiatrists than in any other profession.

One night in 1955 when I was twenty-seven, Karl Abenheimer, then aged over seventy, came round to discuss a problem over a bottle of Tokay. He had a patient in psychotherapy with him. A consultant anaesthetist. This patient had led him to suppose (had told him directly, in so many words) that he had killed three people in the last year, while he had been in therapy, by unobtrusively curtailing their oxygen in the course of long, complex, surgical operations. He kept his overall statistics normal, so that he had no more statistically significant anaesthetic deaths than the average for his sort of job. Anyway, he had had a good run for the last three months so was now about to kill the next victim. He would choose someone with a bad heart, poor lungs, or what not, so that their death would not raise any eyebrows.

Abenheimer had a PhD in law. He had been in analysis with Frieda Fromm-Reichman, at one time married to Eric Fromm. He had studied with Karl Jaspers and had been practising psychotherapy full time for at least twenty-five years. Could this chap simply be having him on? Over the years, all psychiatrists are told some extraordinary stories and it is not always easy to know what to believe, even at the best of times. There is a condition called *pseudologia phantastica* in which the patient elaborates fantastic events and yarns, sometimes very plausible, so that it can be very difficult, impossible to be sure . . .

Nevertheless, Abenheimer had become almost sure (how could he be *absolutely* sure?) that his patient was telling the truth. It was fantasy acted out in fact. Now he was asking himself whether he should do anything. Technically, what he ought to do, and all he ought to do, would be to try to get the patient to see why he was doing what he was doing. A correct psychoanalytic interpretation was the most skilful way to stop all forms of action under the heading of psychopathic, antisocial, acting-out behaviour in someone capable of *realizing* (not 'schizoid insight') its truth. Such a realization could effect a structural mutation of the whole personality.

Anyway, Abenheimer had 'interpreted' to the anaesthetist what he was doing. It did not make any difference. Indeed, the anaesthetist had come along to him to get treatment for just this piece of pathological behaviour.

After a year of treatment, the existential-Jungian-psychoanalytic psychotherapy was not working. Should Abenheimer tell the patient that what he was doing was *wrong* and risk getting confused with his super-ego? Should he refuse to go on seeing him if he did not promise to stop it? Was not his best chance of stopping it not in fact to stay in existential psychotherapy, the aim of which was to help him to realize why he was fulfilling the compulsion about which he was complaining? Should he approach the superintendent of the hospital he worked in? But he was not medically qualified. His patient might well deny it all and brazen it out, putting him, Abenheimer, in a queer position.

So? What would you do? In *his* position? A German-Jewish naturalized refugee without medical qualifications in Glasgow in 1955, talking to an ex-captain RAMC, a young psychiatrist at Glasgow University?

The Department of Psychological Medicine was nick-named the Department of Psycho-Semites because, apart from the professor, the five most senior members of it were Jews.

One of them told me that before he was given the appointment he had a meeting with the Professor:

Rodger: 'You're Jewish, aren't you?'

Freeman: 'Yes.'

'You don't look Jewish, you know what I mean?'

'No.'

'You're not *orthodox*, are you, or anything like that?'

'Oh no.'

'There's no anti-semitism here, you know, so you shouldn't have any problems, you know what I mean?'

'Good, good.'

'No, you shouldn't have any problems. (*Pause.*) You're sure you're not orthodox?'

'Oh no, I'm a psychoanalyst.'

'Oh yes, of course, of course, no you shouldn't have any problems. Just say you're Presbyterian, you know what I mean?'

Through my Jewish friends I attended a lecture given by

Martin Buber to perhaps fifty men at a Jewish Society in Glasgow. I was the only non-Jew present.

Buber was short with unkempt hair and a long white beard – a reincarnation of some Old Testament prophet. I remember distinctly one second of the evening. He was standing at the lectern and had been going on about the human condition, God and the Covenant with Abraham, when suddenly he grasped the large, weighty Bible before him with both hands, raised it as high as possible above his head, smashed it down on the lectern and, standing with his arms outstretched, exclaimed, 'What good is that Book to us, after the Extermination Camps!' He was very angry indeed with God for what He had done to the Jews. And no wonder.

I was still trying to hold together neurology and psychiatry.

The medical department referred a case of multiple sclerosis for a neuropsychiatric report before sending him off to the neurological unit at Killearn.

He was a man in his late thirties, confined for some time already to a wheelchair. He seemed without doubt to be suffering from multiple sclerosis or whatever finer-pointed diagnosis might be made at Killearn; he definitely presented the clinical picture of someone with well-established multiple sclerosis.

Just to see what would happen, I hypnotized him and told him to get up out of his wheelchair and walk. He did – for a few steps. He would have fallen if he had not been supported and helped back to his chair. He might still be walking now if I (and he) had not lost nerve after those first three or four steps – he had not been supposed to be able to walk for over a year.

Multiple sclerosis tends to get worse. But it can stop at any time, often, though not necessarily, to start up its insidious devastation again later.

At any time a sudden, inexplicable, usually very short-lived, partial and, very occasionally, apparently virtual remission of symptoms can occur.

This happened to the cellist, Jacqueline du Pré, who was stricken with multiple sclerosis when she was twenty-eight. A year after she had apparently lost the co-ordination of both her arms forever, she awoke one morning to discover them 'miraculously' all right again. This remission lasted four days, during which time she made several memorable recordings (Chopin and Fauré cello sonatas) without, obviously, having been able to practise the cello for a long time.

One imagines the organic destruction to be irreversible. Yet, even with irreversible organic destruction, function sometimes returns: it seems to be reversible, if only momentarily or for a short time.

If only we could find a way to evoke such 'remissions of symptoms'. But at present scientific medicine has not found the way to generate the phenomena of these 'spontaneous' remissions to therapeutic order.

I think my patient staggered and would have fallen after three or four steps because I lost my nerve. I had not faith so much as a sort of bland assurance, until it happened, and then I had not the faith behind my arrogance to believe that what I saw *was* happening. It must be 'hysterical', I gasped to myself – and that had been the end of that.

I never heard of him taking any steps again and that was the last occasion I ever practised hypnosis in a formal sense. Something happened in me that I still do not know what to make of. I was overcome by a complete taboo. It was not for me. It was not my destiny. But hypnosis remains very important in understanding what I was trying to come to terms with, to find terms for, to give terms to – how we induce others, as others induce us, to believe, perceive, think, feel, and do.

I greatly regretted the professional pressure to specialize *either* in child psychiatry *or* in adult psychiatry. I was very taken by children, especially under the age of five – under the age when I as a child first started to meet other children of my age.

I met at that time one of the most remarkable young chaps I have ever come across.

Rob was brought along by his mother to Notre Dame Child Guidance Clinic in January 1954. He was two years and six months. The clinic's clinical psychologist, mistaking his age for three and a half, gave him an IQ of 131. He was one of the most *intelligent* two-year-olds one is ever likely to meet.

His mother said he had bitten and scratched almost since birth and had become worse since a baby sister was born the year before. She could neither leave Rob alone with his sister, nor let him play with other children. He had bitten a little girl just under one eye. He had never tried to bite his mother, however. Sometimes he screamed.

He came into my room and, without a word, attacked a dolls' house. He pulled the drawers out of a chest-of-drawers, disarranged and upended the beds, disarrayed the furniture. He put sand into a teacup and poured it out several times. He handed me a cup of sand with a saucer. I took it.

'Thank you!' I said, ironically.

'That's not tea, that's *dirt*,' he said, contemptuously.

He went through the same routine a week later. He played with sand.

'I'm playing with dirt. You should be annoyed at me.' I shrugged my shoulders. I wasn't.

One week, when he came, I was not there.

'Mummy didn't want me to come, but I did and you weren't there,' he told me reproachfully the following week. For four months thereafter he shunned me. He played with six or seven other children and a play therapist.

When eventually he came into my room again he asked me to leave him to play by himself, and not to go away.

These two requests seemed to express perfectly what other people wanted in therapy with me. They wanted to enact some sort of drama, with me there but not interfering, not stopping them, or trying to change them by 'making interpretations', hypnosis, or other techniques designed to change them. I was drawn more and more in that direction. With some people, children and adults, the best way to help them out of the *impasse* they seemed to be in, was to help them to enact in my presence the drama that was their particular way to a calmer, more balanced, more integrated, more wholesome, more healthy state of mind. But this drama itself was usually construed as the very pathological process that I was supposed to stop – that is, to cure.

Playing with the dolls' house, Rob yanked the baby doll out of bed and threw it on the floor. He threw the other human figures down the stairs of the house, shouting 'They're all dead.' He repeated this sort of thing again and again. 'Leave me to play with this myself.' 'Don't go away.' Time and again he killed the whole family.

He made up and drew stories. 'Here is a snake, and here is a chimney. The snake bites the chimney and turns into the chimney and a waterfall drowns the snake.'

'This is mummy and daddy in bed – daddy goes to the bathroom – here comes the rain – it covers mummy up – and here is a fire brigade – it puts out the rain with a fire.'

I just let him get on with it.

He took the mummy and the daddy up to the rooftop and placed them on the chimneys. He knocked them together violently and threw them down. Sometimes when he did this only the mummy fell. Sometimes they were both killed. Sometimes only the mummy was killed. Why? 'Because she is naughty to daddy.'

One day he declared that the wee girl was sick, and the goody tucked her into bed. 'The baddy would not be doing this,' he said. 'He would kill her.'

He played at aeroplanes crashing into each other, at trucks crashing into each other. Houses and trucks were bombed by the aeroplanes, which then crashed. He covered over two trucks that had crashed together with sand. He wrecked the hospital and knocked down all the toys in the toy cupboard.

Me: 'You seem to be pretty angry with someone.'

Rob: 'I'm just angry with nobody. I'm just going mad.'

He picked out various animals and asked their names: 'Is this a horse? Is this a cow? Is this a lion?' He took out all the animals, one after the other, in this way. Then he said, 'The goody cowboy is growing strong and the baddy is growing weaker.'

Me: 'How's that?'

Rob: 'He's dead. He fell in the mud, I mean the snow, and he's buried.'

At the end of our last session, two years after we first met, he played at the sand tray with two big ships, a little ship and a red swan. He buried the two big ships in the sand. The little ship comes along, he told me, in the morning and gets them up. Meanwhile the red swan sailed around in the sand 'feeling very happy and pleasant'. Finally they all sailed around together. As they did so, he said: 'You have to listen to the end of this story.' He put a large green tree in the sand. He sailed the two big ships, the little ship and the red swan past the tree. 'The ships don't see it – but they don't bother, they just go past it.'

I said I thought he was going to grow up straight and tall like the tree he had stuck in the sand. He was thoughtful. 'When I grow up I am going to chop down many big trees.' He sailed a little ship round the sand, in and out of the assembled trees and animals – 'and the wee, wee ship sails far away.'

David is a young man of twenty-three. He has been in hospital on two occasions since the age of sixteen and been in psychotherapy with two previous therapists. Clinically, I think that there would be general agreement that he is an ambulatory schizophrenic.

He is heavily muffled in scarves and overcoat; bedraggled, scraggy ends of woollen sleeves; down-at-heel shoes; often very filthy and ill-fitting clothes; unkempt; never takes any of his top clothes off in my presence; tall,

but walks like a half-shut knife, stooping, round-shoul-
dered, deliberately like an old man.

Of his body he says (among other things): 'It just hangs
on me. It seems just a lot of rags of flesh hanging from my
bones. It doesn't particularly belong to me. It feels dead.
It's just like some more clothes. I've no feelings in it.'

He is dissociated from it. *It* doesn't feel alive. *He* doesn't
feel human.

The above quotation is enough, I hope, to establish the
fact that one of his symptoms is a state of depersonalization.
That is the clinical term for how he feels. He himself
complains of this condition. He suffers from it.

In the course of psychotherapy one gradually begins to
discover more about his condition. The ramifications are
endless – here I have to simplify and omit a great deal:

1. One discovers more about the history of his
   relationship to his body.

2. One discovers his relationship with other people,
   particularly their *physical presence*.

3. Meaning, particularly implicit meaning, of the
   fantasy level of his bodily experience and symbolic
   functions relating to his and other people's bodies
   become clearer.

4. Aspects of his experience of himself as a physical
   presence in the world of which he is not aware
   become apparent to both of us; that is, to use a
   psychoanalytic idiom that has become terribly
   misunderstood, unconscious facets become conscious.

5. And, in particular, his physical experience of
   himself in relation to me, in the here and now,
   with all the carry-over, or transference, from his
   past and other experiences in the present outside
   the consulting room, become evident.

6. Finally, in the course of all this exploration, the
   medium on which, and the pivot around which, it

all revolves at all times – our relationship – it
gradually becomes apparent to both of us that the
way he experiences his body is the outcome of
what he is *doing* to his own experience, for reasons
which take some while to figure out, but which
make complete sense once they are brought to
light. In the course of working through all this, the
situation, as he experiences it, becomes quite
radically changed; indeed, to use the idiom of
existential analysis, it is not too much to say that
his whole existence is modified or, to use a
synonymous expression, his whole being-in-the-
world is transformed. He undergoes at least a
partial metamorphosis.

Let me try to summarize some of these developments. I
shall do so without sticking rigidly to the subdivision I have
just given.

We find him at the age of eight or nine becoming
fascinated by Tom Thumb and Pinocchio. He makes little
plasticine figures and buries them. Why? It seems relevant
that he has bilateral undescended testicles, which began to
attract attention – examinations, talk of operations.

He is inordinately afraid of being hit or pinched – he
avoids games, rough-and-tumbles. He is operated on. He
withdraws further from any physical contact with people.
He becomes very conscious of his body as a physical object
isolated in space from other human beings.

In his teens he lives with father. Father's girlfriend –
physically naked – father and girlfriend make love with him
around. Father sometimes loses his temper with him, hits
him: he feels increasingly abject, cowardly, frightened. He
decides to 'agree' to everything. He becomes compliant,
dishonest, insincere, flatters, internally hates, externally
fawns.

He falls into a relationship with his father that is still
going on. To please him, he makes the tea, takes his father's

clothes to the laundry, does the housework. He feels he is
changing into a woman. Is that a delusion or a realization?

Now, taking these sorts of things into consideration,
given all this – the past history of his body, his relationships
with others – consider his present position as he describes it
to me.

He is sitting reading a newspaper on Sunday morning.
His father takes it out of his hand, saying jocularly,
'You've had that long enough,' and sits down imperturb-
ably to read it.

For a split second David feels furious. But, at the same
moment as he imagines himself hitting his father, he
imagines his father brutally hitting him. He feels his testicles retracting in fright. He feels limp, lifeless, helpless.
He manages to make himself offer his father a cup of tea.

Increasingly he experiences 'flashes' of murderous fury
against his father – all at instances of thoughtlessness,
casualness, hypocrisy, imperviousness. He makes his father
a cup of tea and his father just grunts. He could smash cup
and saucer in his face.

His father comes in late at night, bangs the door, wakes
him up. His father sits on a sofa in front of him fondling his
secretary with whom he is having an affair. He feels that he
is treated as a eunuch or as a housemaid or, sometimes, as
his father used to treat his mother.

He feels humiliated and mystified. But he has fawned on
his father for too long. His fury is total, a blind rage. If he
tries to put it into words, he stumbles and becomes choked
with rage, shame, impotence, fear. Besides, his father can
out-match him in words, as well as physically. He cannot
stand his father. He cannot stand himself. He cannot live
with his father. He cannot leave him. Why? He is too 'ill' to
earn more than a few pounds a week as a male char. He is as
frightened to be alone as he is to be with people. He cannot
live with his father and he cannot live with himself. He
cannot live with himself, because he despises himself so
much as a coward, an invalid, a mental cripple, because he

so abjectly wants affection, because his outward manner is an almost total negation of his inner feelings, and so on. He cannot live with his father because if he gives vent to his rage he will either (i) make a fool of himself, (ii) kill his father, (iii) make his father angry so that his father orders him out of the house, or (iv) his father will feel he is getting worse and will stop paying for sessions with me, or (v) his father will hit him as he has done often enough in the past.

From his point of view, from his position in his world as he experiences it, what can he do? What move can he make? If life is unliveable, how can he live in this unliveable situation? He does not kill himself – what are his options? He has taken up several.

One is the construction of a completely imaginary world – a private Utopia inhabited by the 'subterraneous'. He keeps a diary; he writes me long letters that he always asks to have back. He writes trenchantly and, at best, very well.

Instead of killing his father, he understands him. He has an extraordinarily highly developed perceptiveness in certain respects, although much less so about his own life than about mine.

He escapes from himself into a myriad of bits and pieces in fantasy, which come to dead debris floating on a lifeless ocean. He is fascinated by the sort of dashing young man he would like to be. He imagines what delightful young bitches such a young man would fuck. He imagines himself one of these bitches.

He is painfully aware he is not a man and does not feel a man. Instead of being that man, he takes on, or into, himself the bitch that he is fucking. One outcome of this circuit is that his male intellect despises his 'bitchy' feelings, which he is afraid will reveal themselves through his body.

Hence the layers of old men's tattered clothing, as far removed as clothing can be from that of a 'fascinating bitch'. His body: this place of rage, terror, desire and despair. This place of life, which is too harrowing and too fraught with too many conflicts and contradictions that entangle him, that he cannot resolve or transcend. What does he do? He withdraws from his body. He dissociates himself from it. He refuses to *be* it, live it, inhabit it, permeate it with himself. It is not difficult to do this up to a point. Anybody can do it in an armchair with a hand resting on the arm of the chair and play at looking at that arm lying there. What has it to do with me? Look. It's moving. How strange. And so on.

The important point is that he now realizes that he is suffering from depersonalization only in so far as he is depersonalizing himself in a situation in which he finds that he is being depersonalized – that is, simply, not being treated as a person. A condition and a process in which he originally felt himself to be the passive victim is *now* the outcome of his own action on his own experience – that is, of his own *praxis* – in a situation that is for him untenable, *almost* checkmate, except for this move.

Now he very actively feels flooded with anger, then with terror; then there is his own withdrawal from this tidal wave of feeling, leaving his body limp and lifeless.

When Phillip was fourteen he came home from school one day to find his mother lying on her bed in a pool of blood. She had died from a haemoptysis. She had drowned in the blood she had vomited. She had tuberculosis of the lungs. Two months later he came home from school one day to find his father dangling behind the living-room door. He was dead. He had hanged himself.

However, his father had not committed suicide before, in the preceding two months, he had harangued and accused Phillip again and again to the effect that he, Phillip, had caused his mother's death – by being conceived, by exhausting her through pregnancy and his birth and his whole life.

Phillip went to stay with relatives of his mother. Within six months he was admitted to the psychiatric unit of the Glasgow University Department of Psychiatry.

He smelled awful. He was incontinent of urine and faeces, given to staggering and walking peculiarly. He gesticulated in strange ways without speaking, seemed almost completely self-absorbed, and could not care less about his surroundings or the people in them.

Although for the most part silently self-absorbed, there were times when he would appear to be hyper-alert. Then he would start to flutter all over, from head to fingertips and toes, very much like a bird. He had developed a stutter, accompanied by a silent array of complicated involuntary tics: blinks, twitches, fibrillations, darts and flashes of eyes, cheeks, tongue, hands and fingers.

In the course of two months in hospital he was much the same, but had succeeded in antagonizing everyone so much – the other patients and the staff – by his soiling and smell, and, even more, by his total could-not-care-less attitude to them, that they described him as 'cheeky' or 'arrogant'. It was time to transfer him to a mental hospital for long-term care and treatment.

There was no question of the diagnosis. He was an acute (probably becoming chronic) catatonic schizophrenic. When he had anything to say, it was clear that he was hallucinated, very paranoid and very deluded.

He had no brothers and sisters. No relatives to whom he was close. There was literally no one to 'take' him. *No* one who wanted him. The nursing staff wanted to 'get him out' of the ward as soon as possible.

There was indeed something so beyond any decent ordering of things that it is not difficult to understand how he, as the token, as an ugly visible, shitting, smelling reminder of his own story, should be shunned, cut off: that is, *cursed*.

To look, even, at someone as it were *cursed* by the powers that be is to risk being drawn into the orbit of the curse oneself, out of the orbit of the ordinary world, into the obscene. He was obscene.

Perhaps for this reason too his diagnosis was that of

'schizophrenic', when, rationally, it should have been something like an extreme schizophrenoform reaction to catastrophic loss.

He was broken up, shattered to pieces by what had happened. He was staggering. He had been through a literally *staggering* experience. He was *staggered*. He had been struck – not quite *dumb*. He could utter sounds, but nothing coherent came out of his mouth. Just scraps, shreds, drivel, a sudden bellow, a moan, a laugh.

Apart from coming across Phillip in the ward, I saw him alone in my office for about an hour at a time thirty-five times during the six weeks he was in the unit. In other words, I saw him every day.

The reason I did this was that the first time I interviewed him alone, having told the attendant nurse with him to leave, and invited him to have a seat, he sat down and told me a bit about 'where he was at'. He was mainly occupied in pondering the mysteries of the calculus and what actually *was* the lowest common denominator of anything. Most of the time he was out in what I would now call hyperspace. That is, his consciousness, so he told me, was 'spaced out', to use a colloquialism that came in a few years later with the advent of the drug culture. He was out there in the galaxy; there were other intelligences; his mind was bewildered, but in the space in which he was transported most of the time, clarification was coming from the powers that be in reality. This world, the ward, were there, he understood, in some sense, but in a very shadowy sense indeed: as a sort of a shadow of consciousness in the world of 'pure abstraction' – a point he insisted upon. I offered to help him. He accepted my offer. We shook hands and he was conducted back to the ward, where he resumed his usual ward behaviour.

It was only when I was more than halfway through writing up his clinical notes that it dawned on me how extraordinary that interview was and how extraordinary that I could take it so blandly for granted. If there were, then or now, any drug known to world psychiatry that could transform the clinical picture of acute catatonic schizophrenia into the clinical picture of a quiet guy sitting in a chair talking about the calculus, the lowest common denominator, stuff very much along the lines of what John Lilly and others have since written about – consciousness, space, time, different levels of reality – for an hour with no harmful side-effects, its fame and use would have spread round the world. All the more so if it were cheap, quick, painless and harmless. This would be a discovery indeed. Its discoverer would be in the running for a Nobel Prize. Any chemical that could effect such a transformation, even for an hour, even for five minutes, would be heralded as a medico-psychiatric, biochemical, scientific breakthrough of the first order. It could only be the thin end of a wedge. Science would expand and widen out that wedge in not too long a time. Like the early flying-machines: as soon as we knew how to get a machine with a man in it off the ground for a few seconds for a few metres, we were already flying beyond the moon.

I noted at the time about Phillip that 'what is most schizogenic for this boy [and I learned this the hard way] is dishonesty and hypocrisy.'

Phillip generated in *everyone* who came near him mixed feelings of revulsion, at the sight of him and the *smell* of him, and feeling sorry for him, just because he was so repulsive, as well as at his evident misery. The result was that hardly anyone could resist trying to appear to him to be kind and loving, but fleeing out of sight and smell of him as quickly as possible – not because they could not stand him, but for some other necessity.

I thought that as soon as I caught on to my own mixed feelings and got over my embarrassment that I did not want to smell his shit at all, a lot of the haze he was in seemed to clear up. In clinical, psychiatric terms, being straight and candid to him within an overall attitude of benevolence (I felt very sorry for his plight and very much wanted to help him, if possible) seemed to produce a remarkable temporary remission of symptoms.

This observation, like the others I have mentioned along similar lines, says nothing about whether Phillip was suffering from an illness of some kind, or about the as yet unascertained micro-molecular events going on in his central nervous system. But again it seems very relevant to the way we treat people in Phillip's predicament.

True, as he sat on the chair, there were a few twitches, twinges, a few flutters. But, thank God, he did not piss and shit in my office. He never did. Nevertheless, what he talked about the first time, and later – such things as prehistoric clairvoyance, problems of the infinitely small, interplanetary visitations floating as a sort of mist of consciousness in interstellar space – would be taken by many, probably almost all, psychiatrists today as the very epitome of psychotic ideation, however it is subclassified.

Worse still, from this psychiatric point of view, he sometimes found the ward space to be like a sphere in which he was a pin in the centre. This was one reason he was staggering so much. Because in the spherical spaceship he was in, which we saw as a rectangular ward, he had not learned to walk steadily. Even if he had learned to walk steadily in his sphere, how does an infinitely small dot 'walk'?

Besides, there was a man he never saw behind his bed at night. Abstractions would move. An abstract triangle would torment him from a corner. He sometimes heard a black man's voice, but he could not make out what it was saying.

Two shocking experiences such as he went through in two months lend credibility to calling his schizophreniform psychosis 'reactive'. Maybe there is a straw that will break any camel's back. Not everyone reacts to most horrific experiences with a psychotic reaction. A psychotic reaction is psychotic but a reaction nonetheless; even an intelligible reaction, but psychotic nonetheless.

If Phillip had kept up a policy of 'love me, love the smell of my shit', neither my wife nor I, nor anyone – his concerned social worker, a foster family – nor drugs nor any other therapy, then or now, could have done anything for him – I do not think.

Presumably both his parents had been psychotic. Ergo, very poor prognosis.

I thought that if he were consigned to a mental hospital aged fourteen (there was no 'adolescent' unit) however poor his prognosis, this could only make it worse. Indeed, he would probably be finished for life.

He came to stay with us – my wife Anne and me and three children under four.

Everything went incredibly well from the start. His incontinence stopped almost completely from the moment he came to stay with us and within a couple of weeks he was shaking but not staggering. He spoke falteringly but coherently. After three months he was sufficiently together again, and we arranged for him to stay with another family, a foster-family arrangement fixed up by one of the department's psychiatric social workers.

It was glaringly obvious to me that the success of the venture all hinged on his relation to Anne. She is one of the least emotionally hypocritical people I have ever met and has very little patience with it in others. She gave him very little to go crazy about on that score and she did not let him get away with that sort of thing on his part. So they got on very well.

We last met him fifteen years later, when he came to see us to tell us about himself. He was married, had two children, had a steady job and was taking evening classes in psychology.

When I was working in my first university appointment in Glasgow, the newly set-up interview rooms had just been built and each room had its desk and chair, and two armchairs at a lower level for the patient and a possible other person with the patient. For my psychiatric interviews I moved from the chair behind the desk to the armchair in front of the desk at the same level as the patient's chair.

One day I was called to the professor's office.

'I hear, Ronnie, that you see patients in front of your desk. Is that right?'

'Yes, sir.'

'I know you are very interested in patients but I just want to warn you – don't get too close to them.'

I gave a seminar to the senior staff of a psychiatric unit in a sophisticated general hospital in London. Patients were excluded routinely, without question of course, from all staff meetings and from this meeting in particular because what might 'come up' would be too 'sensitive' for them. All junior staff, whether psychiatrists, nurses, psychiatric social workers, psychologists or students were also excluded.

After I had talked for a while about how a psychiatric diagnosis can affect our relations with the patient, the chief psychiatric social worker asked if she could put a question to me.

'Dr Laing, I am told that you allow your schizophrenic patients to talk to you.'

'Yes, I do,' I replied.

You could have heard a pin drop – but no pin dropped.

In this unit it is regarded as improper to encourage patients in whom a schizophrenic process is active to 'verbalize', especially if their 'verbalizations' are strewn with schizophrenic symptomatology. That is why they were being given drugs – to inhibit, suppress, repress, to stop as effectively and as precisely as possible the schizophrenic biochemical processes. To encourage 'verbalization' would be to go in the opposite direction. Why give drugs to inhibit the process and encourage its freeing through 'verbalization' at the same time? It is like fanning a fire to life at the same time as trying to blow it out.

In this unit all psychiatric social-work students have a

standing order not to permit any schizophrenic patient in
the wards to talk to them.

In a recent seminar that I gave to a group of psychoanalysts,
my audience became progressively aghast when I said that I
might accept a cigarette from a patient without making an
interpretation. I might even offer a patient a cigarette. I
might even give him or her a light.

'And what if a patient asked you for a glass of water?' one
of them asked, almost breathlessly.

'I would give him or her a glass of water and sit down in
my chair again.'

'Would you not make an interpretation?'

'Very probably not.'

A lady exclaimed, 'I'm totally lost.'

I met Paul Tillich several times in Glasgow in 1955 and
1956. He went pretty far over the edge for some. I remember sitting beside a dear old devout Protestant Glaswegian
lady at one of his lectures, when he started to get his teeth
into this passage from Mark's Gospel:

27. And Jesus went out, and his disciples, into the
    towns of Caesarea Philippi: and by the way he
    asked his disciples, saying unto them, Whom do
    men say that I am?

28. And they answered, John the Baptist: But some
    say, Elias; and others, One of the prophets.

29. And he saith unto them, But whom say ye that I
    am? And Peter answereth and saith unto him,
    Thou art the Christ.

30. And he charged them that they should tell no
    man of him.

Who do men say that I am?

Maybe He did not know Himself? Maybe at that moment
in His career He did not yet know who He was. Maybe He

never knew. If Christ was Jesus, very God of very God verily incarnated as Man in Man, *a* man with a human body – and a human mind – maybe He could not know who He was. That is specifically, individually and categorically, generically, we may or may not know or think or believe or hope we are all sons and daughters of God; and if we are, which? The human mind *has* to ask 'Who, what, whence, whither, why am I?' And it is very doubtful if the human mind can answer any of these questions.

Perhaps Paul Tillich went too far.

He doubted, even, when Jesus asked His disciples who He was, whether He knew Himself. Maybe He had no idea Himself who He was, and was genuinely interested in hearing their views.

The old lady sitting beside me turned to me when the lecture was over, almost crying, and said, 'It's not fair for a man like that to come here and destroy the faith of an old woman like me.'

Postscript

When I left Glasgow to take up a job at the Tavistock Clinic and to undergo four years of training at the Institute of Psychoanalysis, it was becoming clearer to me where my interest lay. It had to do with mental misery. What were the necessary or sufficient conditions to occasion mental misery of any kind? More particularly, what caused the sort or sorts of mental misery with which I was being trained to deal, to 'treat', as a psychiatrist in the UK? More particularly still, I had begun to get into focus the domain of interplay between what happens within and between people.

Then, as now, only what mainstream psychiatrists called the lunatic fringe of the psychiatric profession spent much time listening to psychiatric patients, or much time in their company one way or another. Whatever else was going on in psychiatry, it was, and is, one interface in the socio-economic–political structure of our society where camaraderie, solidarity, companionship, communion is almost impossible, or completely impossible. Psychiatrists and patients were, and are, too often ranged on opposite sides. Before we meet, we are far apart.

The psychiatrist-patient rift across the sane-mad line seemed to play a part in some of the misery and disorder occurring within the field of psychiatry. Maybe this loss of human camaraderie was the most important thing. Maybe its restoration was the *sine qua non* of 'treatment'.

What does what goes on between people contribute to the sort of misery a psychiatrist is expected to 'treat'? The misery of a person in extreme mental misery is usually

apparently related to their relations with other human
beings. Indeed, we sometimes almost take it for granted
that most people seem to go on most about their relations
with others.

It is taken as an established clinical fact that people
deemed to be suffering from most forms of mental illness
find it difficult, if not impossible, to form ordinary bonds
with ordinary other people, and vice versa. Occasionally a
'remission', at least a partial remission, may occur, and I
saw dozens of remissions one New Year's morning. Why
did dozens of remissions not occur every day of the year?

I wanted to see further and more clearly what direct
personal communication is. Could an understanding of
communication, miscommunication, non-communication
and excommunication contribute to the problems of Western psychiatry?

In this book I have been trying to show a way to see what
I am describing so that what I am trying to describe can be
seen. The personal area tends to be ignored by most
psychiatrists. Why? Professionals, I think, fear it as much
as patients. Psychiatry tries to be as scientific, impersonal
and objective as possible towards what is most personal and
subjective. The disordered suffering treated by psychiatrists has to do with what are our most personal and private
thoughts and desires. No other branch of medicine has to
contend with this domain so much. Nothing whatever in
Western medical training exists to adapt students and
young doctors to integrating the personal aspect into clinical theory and practice. The result is that when doctors are
faced with this inner suffering, they are disoriented, insofar
as they refer themselves back to their conventional training
for orientation.

By the time this memoir ends I was thirty years old and
had written my first book, *The Divided Self*. I knew what I
wanted to address myself to for the foreseeable future in
theory and in practice. I began to focus on this personal
factor. You and me.

Notes

1. Myerson, A. in Hill, D., *The Politics of Schizophrenia*, University Press of America, New York and London.
2. Hirschman, J., *Antonin Artaud Anthology*, City Lights Books, San Francisco, 1965, p. 135.
3. Buber, M., *I and Thou* (trans. W. Kaufmann), T. & T. Clark, Edinburgh, 1970.
4. Haley, J., *Reflections on Therapy and Other Essays*, The Family Therapy Institute of Washington, 1981, p. 158.
5. Henderson, D. K. and Gillespie, R. D., *A Text-Book of Psychiatry*, Oxford University Press, 1927.
6. Schorstein, J., *The Metaphysics of the Atom Bomb*, The Philosophical Journal, Vol. 1, No. 1, pp. 33–46.
7. Jaspers, K., *General Psychopathology*, Manchester University Press, 1962.
8. Laing, R. D., *The Facts of Life*, Penguin, 1976, pp. 115–16.